STUTTERING
SOLVED

D1569065

Martin F. Schwartz, Ph.D.

STUTTERING
SOLVED

 McGraw-Hill Book Company

New York · St. Louis · San Francisco · Bogota · Düsseldorf
Madrid · Mexico · Montreal · Panama · Paris
São Paulo · Tokyo · Toronto

Copyright © 1976 by Martin F. Schwartz.

All rights reserved. Printed in the United States of America. No part of this publication may be reproduced, stored in a retrieval system, or transmitted, in any form or by any means, electronic, mechanical, photocopying, recording, or otherwise, without the prior written permission of the publisher.

First McGraw-Hill Paperback Edition, 1977

Reprinted by arrangement with J. B. Lippincott Company.

1234567890MU MU783210987

Library of Congress Cataloging in Publication Data

Schwartz, Martin F   1936–
  Stuttering solved.

  Includes index.
  1. Stuttering. I. Title.
[RC424.S38   1977]   616.8′554   77–4175
ISBN 0–07–055753–5

To Judy

Contents

CONTENTS

PART II
THE TREATMENT

PART III
CASE HAPPENINGS

PART IV
SUGGESTIONS FOR
HELPING STUTTERERS

Foreword

MY ATTEMPT TO UNDERSTAND stuttering, which had long been an enigma for speech therapists, was sparked serendipitously by the unusual speech behavior of a four-year-old child whom I encountered while working as a consultant at the New York University Medical Center. At that time I was a professor of speech science at another university, engaged in basic research in human communication, but I had also been trained as a clinician in speech correction and now the challenge of solving the clinical problem of stuttering seemed much more relevant than my work as a speech scientist.

This book describes the new treatment I developed for stuttering, based on a theory that explains, for the first time, why people stutter. The success rates for my patients and those of the therapists whom I have trained in this new method of treatment range between 83 and 92 percent, three times greater than has heretofore been demonstrated for any other method. It was my discovery of the physical cause of the stuttering block that enabled me to develop a relatively simple treatment that succeeds in such a high percentage of cases.

My quest for the understanding of stuttering is recounted in the first part of this book. It is written as it happened—as an adventure.

After I was able to account for stuttering in a comprehensive way, I started to treat patients. How the therapy developed and was gradually modified to work for the wide range of apparently dissimilar types of stuttering is told in the second part of the book. Part III presents case histories that illustrate a fascinating variety of stuttering behaviors, introducing the general public to a subculture they may not have known existed. The book ends with advice for the parents of stutterers, for teachers with stuttering children in their classroom, and for the adult stutterer himself.

My purpose in writing this book, which contains my first formal presentation of both theory and therapy, is to put an end to stuttering. Since my intention is to give the interested layman a clear picture of stuttering, the book has no scholarly references. I suspect the book will be controversial as its claims may seem extravagant, but I am willing to demonstrate the therapy with patients at any time. I welcome anyone interested in observing these techniques to come and do so. Treatment programs are now in the process of development throughout the country, and it seems likely that the therapy will be routinely available for the two million American adult stutterers. It is my hope that stuttering as a clinical problem in the United States will become extinct within the near future.

PART I
The Understanding

1
THE RIDDLE
OF
STUTTERING

I ONCE TREATED a child who could release herself from a stuttering block only by pulling a hair out of her head. Though she was only seven, she appeared to be going bald.

Another patient could speak without stuttering only when he tossed a pencil into the air each time he started a sentence; a pen would not do—it had to be a pencil.

One adolescent patient could not speak while standing since the violent backward thrusts of his head invariably caused him to lose his balance and fall. And another youngster, when trying to say his name, would tense, gasp, shake his body, stamp his foot, and then finally slap his face before saying the word.

What made stutterers struggle so violently? And how was it possible for them in the very next moment to whisper or sing the same words effortlessly?

Why didn't they stutter when they were alone and talked aloud to themselves, or when talking to animals, or when using an assumed accent? Why did a priest I once treated stutter only in the pulpit, an actress only when auditioning, and a mathematician only when discussing formulas?

If it was "nerves" as some thought, why did they never stutter when they were angry? If there was something wrong with their speech, why didn't they stutter all the time?

Stuttering is an affliction that has plagued man since earliest times: the Egyptians had a hieroglyphic for it. There are now more than two million adult stutterers in the United States for whom the simplest act of communication—introducing oneself to strangers, speaking up in a group, even ordering food in a restaurant—can become a nightmare.

In the pages that follow, I propose, for the first time, a solution to this perplexing disorder. I describe the discovery of a *physical cause* of stuttering and give the details of a therapy which has proved successful with a high percentage of patients, both children and adults.

But first, let me describe how it was that I became interested in this problem.

2
A VIEW
FROM THE EMPIRE STATE
OBSERVATORY

IN 1969 I WAS HELPING a surgeon design an operation to improve the speech of children born with cleft palate, an absence of a portion of the roof of the mouth which results in direct communication between nose and mouth. Surgeons would correct this defect, but in about half the cases, speech would not develop normally. The problem was that, although the palate was closed, it was too short to reach the back throat wall, and as a result sound and air would go through the nose whenever speech was attempted. The patient sounded nasal and many of the consonants were unclear.

One day I saw a four-year-old child with this problem who had been fitted with a speech bulb, a piece of plastic attached by orthodontic bands to the teeth, and designed to fill the gap between the palate and the throat. In this case, the speech bulb had a curious effect upon the child's speech. When she wore the bulb her speech was clear—free of nasality and with precisely articulated consonants—but she stuttered. Without the bulb her speech was nasal and unclear—but the stuttering was absent. The question was, why?

I noticed that the stuttering appeared only on certain consonants, sounds which required the buildup of air pressure in the mouth. I knew that when the bulb was out she could not build up much air pressure since the air escaped through the nose. Could stuttering, I wondered, be somehow related to air pressure, perhaps triggered by it?

I had a duplicate bulb made. I drilled a tiny hole through it so that a small amount of air would escape when she spoke. Nothing happened; her speech remained unchanged. I increased the size of the hole to let more air escape so that less air pressure would build up in the mouth—and then, suddenly, a threshold was reached at a certain size opening and the stuttering stopped.

My suspicions were now strongly aroused. If it was air pressure that was triggering the stuttering, and if I could somehow substantially drop the pressure environment in which this young child spoke, the pressure receptors in her lungs would not respond and her stuttering would cease. What I needed to test the theory was the rarefied atmosphere of a mountaintop.

We walked the four blocks from my office to the Empire State Building and took the elevator to the observation tower. Along the way, she had been stuttering because she was wearing the bulb that had been made for her originally. But at the top of the Empire State Building her speech was fluent—without a trace of a stutter.

20

3
THE FLARING
NOSTRILS

I DID NOT THEN START to do therapy at the top of the Empire State Building. Indeed, it was to be three years before I was to do any therapy at all with stutterers. I spent the time, instead, trying to understand the relationship between air pressure and stuttering, and why it was that when I brought adults who stuttered to the top of the building, they still stuttered. What was different?

The answer was slow to emerge.

After the incident with the four-year-old, I spent several weeks observing stuttering children. The more children I observed, the more impressed I was with the variety of behaviors they exhibited; there were about as many types of stuttering, I thought, as there were children who stuttered.

The literature on childhood stuttering was not of much help. The textbooks distinguished between two forms: primary stuttering, characterized by some sort of effortless repetition and prolongation of sound, and secondary stuttering, associated with obvious struggle. This distinction didn't satisfy me since it didn't explain the variety of behavior I was seeing.

Was there a common factor to be found in all of this? Some sort of unifying principle? I made detailed observations of each child, but the more data I amassed, the more variety I observed. Later, when examining my notes—which had grown dismayingly extensive—I discovered that I had made a similar comment about a number of the children.

It was most often expressed this way: "Just before they stuttered their nostrils flared."

After examining more stuttering children, paying careful attention to their nostrils, I observed that if the nostrils flared before the child stuttered they did so invariably and one could predict when the child would stutter by simply looking at his nose.

Other young stuttering children showed none of the flaring, but when I rested a finger against their nostrils, I often felt a tensing just before the onset of stuttering.

The question was, what did the nose, essentially a respiratory organ, have to do with speech and, more particularly, with stuttering?

I brought this question with me to Armonk, a small community some forty miles north of New York City to which my wife and I retreat on weekends. As we drove up the driveway, we were greeted by Brandy, the neighbor's golden retriever, carrying a small branch in his mouth and wagging his tail furiously.

He accompanied us into the house and dropped the branch immediately when my wife offered him a dog biscuit. After devouring it as if he hadn't eaten in a month, he curled up on the dining-room floor and went to sleep.

It was then I noticed that his nostrils flared rhythmically as he breathed. But was the air going in or out of the nostrils when they flared?

I bent over and placed my finger directly in front of his nostrils—in the path of the airstream. The answer became obvious. There was no flow of air when they flared. The flare occurred only prior to inhalation, as if the nose opened to accept the air. And, indeed, that's exactly what was happening.

Watching the nostrils of my normal-speaking neighbors while they talked and when they were silent, I observed no motion at all. That night I paid close attention to my wife as she slept. Again, no nostril flaring.

Lying in bed that night I remembered something I had once learned. In an earlier geological age, amphibians, who were our remote ancestors, could voluntarily open or close their nostrils depending upon whether they were on land or in water. And when they finally became land-based, the muscles that opened the nostrils became vestigial as a cartilage framework was established to keep them open continuously.

Brandy is a retriever, a breed of water-loving dogs, obviously possessing a more prominent development of these ancient muscles. Those stuttering children who displayed nasal flaring probably also had prominently developed nostril muscles.

The following day a friend visited me and we spent

the afternoon in my shop doing carpentry work. We were using a table saw, making a lot of dust, and he sneezed several times. After the first sneeze, I noticed he took in a great deal of air prior to each subsequent one and that prior to the taking in of this air, his nostrils flared.

It was now obvious to me. What I was observing was a reflex. It manifested itself in adults only when there was a sudden need for a substantial amount of air. Given this premise, I now found that the flaring occurred on many occasions: before a yawn, a cough, a sigh, and in the anticipation of any vigorous and sustained physical activity. It seemed to open the breathing passages—to widen them—so that air could enter more easily. Hence, I named it the Airway Dilation Reflex.

4
THE HUNT
FOR THE
REFLEX

THERE ARE OTHER STRUCTURES besides the nostrils involved in the airway. At the office the following Monday morning, I made a drawing of the movable parts of the upper airway (the distance from the nostrils to the vocal cords). The drawing looked like this:

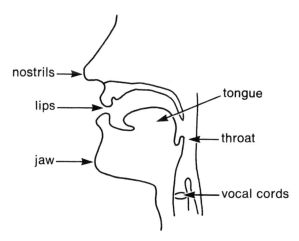

My challenge was clear: to find evidence in the scientific literature which showed that these structures participated actively in the dilation of the airway prior to inhalation.

I walked the short distance to the library of the New York University Medical Center, descended to the stacks, and began my search.

I decided to start with the larynx, the structure that contains the vocal cords. I knew that the space between the cords was the smallest along the airway and I thought, therefore, it might be a sensitive indicator of the presence of a reflex.

My search did not take long. I found that the vocal cords did, indeed, open slightly before each inhalation and close slightly before each exhalation. I discovered that the opening was due to the active contraction of a single pair of muscles, and that the closing was due to the relaxation of these muscles. I found that this observation had been made as early as 1850 and could be found repeatedly in the literature since then.

I began to look for evidence for other structures. The going got tough. There were certainly many reports of the functioning of these structures, but only in relation to such irrelevant activities as chewing or swallowing.

I developed the habit of going to an article that related to a structure, scanning it quickly for its relevance to breathing, then checking its bibliography to see if there were likely leads. If I found one, I would go to it immediately, examine it, and also check its bibliography, which, in turn, led me elsewhere. I was looking for pieces to a puzzle in a veritable sea of pieces.

While reading one of these articles, I came upon a reference to another that had been published in a small, obscure journal. I was in luck as the library subscribed to the journal, and I soon discovered that a large muscle in the tongue contracts just prior to inhalation and relaxes just after it. The action of this muscle served to draw the back of the tongue away from the throat and thereby to dilate it. I thus had evidence of the tongue's participation in the Airway Dilation Reflex.

I now proceeded to research the throat literature and found something which was to be of extreme importance later in the development of my thinking: that the throat of an infant is extremely short, narrow, and flexible and, on occasion, can be subject to kinking—like a garden hose. To combat this, the muscles of the throat are constantly being stimulated to dilate and such stimulation can become enhanced where there is a possibility of imminent kinking.

I wondered, when reading this, if a failure of such muscles to contract might not be the cause of "crib death," a mysterious disorder which kills thousands of infants each year. This possibility was intriguing, and there was some evidence in support of it, but I was committed to solving the riddle of stuttering, and shelved further consideration of this topic for another time.

Although I discovered that the muscles of the throat were under constant stimulation, I was never to find direct evidence of a dilation prior to quiet inhalation. I did, however, discover that the throat muscles in adults actively widen the throat prior to vigorous inhalations, and

27

this was consistent with what I had observed for the nostrils of normal-speaking adults.

So, too, was the evidence for the jaw and lips—no tendency to open during quiet inhalations, but always a dilation during vigorous ones.

I concluded that the Airway Dilation Reflex is fully present before vigorous inhalations—all structures dilate. In addition, both the tongue and vocal cords show dilation prior to quiet inhalations, with the vocal cords exhibiting greater movement than the tongue. The vocal cords are apparently the most sensitive indicators (have the lowest threshold of excitation) of all the structures involved in the Airway Dilation Reflex.

It was possible to determine whether the Airway Dilation Reflex was occurring in those children whose nostrils flared before they stuttered. In my laboratory, I had a machine designed to indicate whether the vocal cords were open or closed. Called a glottograph, it is a sort of miniature radio transmitter and receiver. The transmitter is placed on one side of the child's neck and the receiver on the other. When the vocal cords are closed, a tone, emanating from the transmitter, travels through the cords and is picked up at the receiver. When the vocal cords are open, there is an air gap between them, and the transmitted signal traverses the gap weakly. Thus, if the tone is loud, the vocal cords are closed, and if it is soft, they are open.

I examined several children, all under the age of five, and stuttering with minimal effort. The results were clear: the vocal cords frequently opened prior to each stuttering instance, and this always occurred at the same time the nostrils flared. Here, then, was the confirmatory evidence I was looking for: nostril flaring was an indication of the occurrence of the Airway Dilation Reflex in young stuttering children.

5
AIR PRESSURE
AS A
TRIGGER

W HAT DID THE Airway Dilation Reflex have to do
with stuttering? Why was the reflex occurring at all?
What function did it serve?

The literature on stuttering offered firm evidence
that stuttering emerged in children most often when they
were attempting to speak under conditions of stress.
Stuttering appeared initially after an illness or a trauma
like being bitten by a dog, or moving to a new city or
starting school, and it occurred most frequently when
the child was excited or was trying to get a word in
edgewise. It seemed that stress somehow was provoca-
tive and that the reflex emerged in response to it.

Since the reflex obviously could serve no useful purpose under such conditions, I concluded that its appearance was a mistake, a reflex which somehow manifested
itself inappropriately under the influence of stress.

There is, of course, considerable precedence for
this. For example, in a young child the distention of the
bladder triggers a reflex that empties it. As part of the

socialization process, the maturing child becomes toilet-trained; he learns to inhibit this reflex in all but certain situations. But let the child experience unusual stress and this inhibitory control is temporarily lost and he urinates inappropriately. The pattern is part of the general principle that learned inhibitory controls can be lost under stress.

But what inhibitory control was being lost for the young stutterer? Why was the Airway Dilation Reflex being activated to begin with? What was triggering it?

And then I remembered my experiment with the four-year-old child in the Empire State Building and the conclusion I had drawn. It was air pressure that was triggering the reflex.

But why? What would the air pressure signal? I thought about that for a good while, looked over my notes, and then remembered what I had read about the tendency for a child's throat to kink. If the Airway Dilation Reflex acts as a sort of protective mechanism for the infant's breathing apparatus, then when a kink did form, the reflex would be called into play to deal with it. In this case, the reflex would fire because as the child attempted to exhale against the kink, the pressure in the lungs would suddenly increase—and the pressure receptors within the lungs would start the reflex going.

This seemed a highly plausible theory, which gained strength when I added another piece of information to it: when one speaks there is always an obstruction in the airway. The speech structures establish this obstruction

31

because there must be a buildup of air pressure to make sound. Air pressure in the lungs is the driving force behind speech.

In other words, speech requires air pressure, and, as part of the maturation process, the young child learns to inhibit the firing of the Airway Dilation Reflex in response to it. It was this loss of inhibitory control which I was witnessing in the flaring nostrils of the young stuttering children. Under stress, their brains were misinterpreting the buildup of air pressure required for speech as being the result, not of the attempt to speak, but rather of a life-threatening airway obstruction—a kink—and the reflex emerged automatically.

6
THE REFLEX
AND THE
VOCAL CORDS

I NEXT ADDRESSED MYSELF to the question, was the dilation reflex responsible for stuttering, and, if so, how?

I imagined what would happen if I attempted to speak when the reflex occurred. I sat in my office and uttered a long ah-h-h-h. While making the sound, I envisioned the reflex taking hold of my speaking apparatus: my throat enlarging, the back of my tongue moving forward, without affecting the sound until I opened my vocal cords—and then, there was silence, no sound, only the quiet flow of air from my mouth.

I tried to reconstruct what must happen in the young child who stutters. When he gets set to speak, his vocal cords are brought together gently and then the buildup of air pressure sets them vibrating. But since he is under stress his brain makes a mistake; it misinterprets the build-up of air pressure as the result of a kink, the reflex fires, the vocal cords open wide, and the child becomes temporarily speechless.

What would I do, I wondered, if I suddenly found myself in this predicament? Would I try to talk in a whisper, thus keeping my vocal cords open all the time, or would I try to get sound going somehow? The odds are I would try the latter. And to do so it would be necessary to bring my vocal cords together. But if I did this gently, the firing of the reflex would open them. So why not voluntarily bring them together strongly—before speaking—before the buildup of air pressure and the resultant reflex? And if I brought them together strongly enough, when the reflex did fire, it might not be able to open them, and then maybe I could get some sound going.

But I was not aware of the fact that the muscles that close the cords are much stronger than the muscles that open them. And so what I was learning to do was to lock my cords. Now I could not speak because I had set my cords together too tightly. I had gone from one predicament to another.

Later I was to call this response a conditioned laryngospasm, "conditioned" meaning learned, and "laryngospasm" meaning locking, or excessive tensing, of the vocal cords. I was to discover that this was the heart of the stuttering problem and that all the struggling I observed in stuttering was in reaction to it.

However, I was not to discover this for some time— and not before I had obtained additional facts showing that the laryngospasm was actually the cause of stuttering.

7
PHYSICAL FACTORS
IN
STUTTERING

THERE WAS CERTAINLY no shortage of data from research on stuttering. Much of it pointed to a physical cause that was very likely inherited. For example, a study done many years ago investigated the relationship between twinning and stuttering. Hundreds of pairs of twins were examined and the results showed that among monozygotic (identical) twins, if one twin stuttered, the odds were over 90 percent that the other would, while among dizygotics (fraternal), if one stuttered the odds were under 7 percent that the other would. Here was a disparity far too great to be accounted for by anything else but common genetic inheritance.

Also there were many studies that showed a stuttering incidence, regardless of culture, of about four times more males than females. Here was another fact that could be explained only in terms of some sex-linked inherited factor.

Among the many studies that examined brain-wave patterns in both stutterers and nonstutterers, the majority showed significant differences between the two groups. The fact that such differences could not generally be explained was not important; what was important was that they tended to demonstrate the strong likelihood of a physical factor present in stuttering.

Other statistics strengthened the impression of an inherited factor involved in stuttering. For example, about three quarters of all adult stutterers reported that someone in their family stuttered or had done so at one time. This was fully seven and a half times greater than the incidence of nonstutterers with a stutterer in their families.

Another piece of evidence that localized this physical factor to the vocal cords was based on an unfortunate circumstance. When stutterers underwent an operation for the removal of their vocal cords because of cancer, and subsequently learned a new form of sound production, their speech was invariably stutter-free.

Other facts that pointed to the vocal cords as the source of the difficulty were the well-known observations that stuttering stopped when the patient sang or mouthed his words silently, and was much reduced when he whispered, spoke in a breathy voice, or changed his pitch appreciably.

But these facts, convincing as they were, would not impress the psychiatrists. In order to understand stuttering, I had to take into account the psychiatrists' observations of stutterers.

8
PSYCHOLOGICAL
FACTORS IN
STUTTERING

IMAGINE, IF YOU WERE a psychiatrist, a stutterer coming to you for help and reporting that he stuttered on the "t" sound in the word "to" but never in the words "too" or "two." What would you think?

Or how could you explain the behavior of a male stutterer in his mid twenties who invariably greeted young women by closing his eyes, standing on his toes, grunting, and sticking his tongue out?

Psychiatrists have offered such explanations of stuttering as these:

"Stuttering is caused by the fear of the ego being overwhelmed by the all-powerful autoeroticism. . . . It is a form of gratification of the original oral libido which continues as a postnatal gratification in talking. . . ."

"Stuttering is a pregenital conversion [hysterical] neurosis in that the early problems dealing with the retention and expulsion of the feces have been displaced upward into the sphincters of the mouth. . . ."

"Stuttering represents the act of nursing at an illusory nipple. . . ."

Freud, himself, tried to treat stuttering but was unsuccessful. According to psychiatrists, the problem is clearly deep-seated; it emerges early, usually between three and seven years of age, and can persist throughout life.

Sometimes the onset could be pinpointed, such as after shifting handedness, or starting at a new school, or being bitten by a dog. But still, even with such knowledge, treatment was difficult.

So the psychiatrists concentrated on the symptoms, and on the patients' attitudes toward them. Attempts were made to make patients less anxious about their problem, more accepting of it and more relaxed in general —and, as a result, they sometimes improved and in rare cases even became fluent.

Psychiatrists also tried tranquilizers, hypnosis, electroconvulsive shock therapy, and antispasmodic drugs— all with limited success.

There was no lack of interest. Everyone agreed that anxiety or stress of some sort was the precipitating factor in every stuttering block. Everyone agreed because every adult stutterer said so.

9
THE STRESS
CONNECTION

THE PROBLEM WAS, what caused the stress? Was it, as the psychiatrists suggested, the result of deep-seated unresolved conflicts? Or was it, as some psychologists felt, a set of responses learned in specific contexts and triggered by them?

The two opinions were markedly different. The former held that the elimination of stuttering was basically tied to the resolution of conflict; the latter contended that the solution was dependent upon the learning of new habits.

I decided to ask patients what they felt to be the source of their stress. Many of them had had a variety of psychotherapies, and most reported that, apart from enabling them to adjust better to their problem, the psychotherapy had not improved their speech. They seemed, as a group, to be reasonably well-adjusted and this impression coincided with the research studies that had shown no difference between stutterers and nonstutterers in terms of psychological profile.

None of the stutterers I questioned felt that there was any deep-seated psychological cause for their problem. Most of them were emphatic about this. And I often received an equally emphatic answer to another question, a question posed this way: "Suppose you woke up tomorrow morning with total amnesia. You remembered absolutely nothing about yourself, your past, your environment, even your name. Would you stutter?" The answer given most often was, "Of course not."

It came down to this. If adult stutterers couldn't predict where they would stutter, they wouldn't stutter at all. It was a matter of conscious awareness, not subconscious ordination. They could feel the block coming. They could feel it in their breathing, in a tightness in their chest, their throat, their face, and often in an uncontrollably rampant heartbeat.

And they were rarely mistaken: if they felt they were going to stutter, they did. And the reverse was equally true. If they felt they weren't going to stutter, they virtually never did.

Most stutterers made good use of this ability to predict their blocks. They almost always scanned ahead, sometimes as many as four or five sentences ahead, looking for words with which they might have difficulty, and shifting the conversation to avoid them. They developed the art of word substitution to a high degree; their use of synonyms was thesauruslike. The friends of such a stutterer usually don't know he stutters; they merely think that he sometimes expresses himself in novel language.

40

But this hunting for word substitutes to avoid the stuttering block is very tiring. It makes normal conversation difficult. If the listeners knew the active scanning and mental gymnastics taking place in these seemingly effortless and inconsequential conversations, they would be incredulous.

Much later I was to treat several patients with this form of the problem. They visited me secretively. Hearing about my work with stutterers, they had summoned up the courage to call and confess their predicament. Could I help them with no one knowing? Would they have to stutter in order for me to treat them? Did I have to have their home telephone numbers?

One such patient told me an interesting story. He was a judge in a state court. He had substituted one word for another successfully for years, and his use of language, while sometimes unusual, was nevertheless attractive, and added to his charisma. But he had a problem. He had been offered a federal district judgeship, wanted the post desperately, but couldn't accept it. The reason was that, while he was allowed to paraphrase the charge to the jury in the state court, no such latitude was allowed in the federal court. He would have to read the charge word for word, with no substitutions or circumlocutions, and therefore could not take the job.

When I told him he would have to stutter in order to be treated, he balked. Try as I might, this man was not about to give up his deeply entrenched avoidance patterns. He left and, to my knowledge, still holds the state job.

41

Others, however, were less resistant. Apparently the pain and effort of constantly scanning and avoiding was so great that they overcame their resistance to stuttering and allowed it to happen, thereby learning to prevent it. Once the patient knew he had an acceptable technique for aborting his blocks, he substituted this technique for the less acceptable one of avoiding them. The process was learned quickly, and all that his friends, family, and associates ever realized afterward was that the patient made a lot more sense when he talked.

So it was that I discovered that not every stutterer stutters and that the fear of stuttering could be as real and as devastating as the block itself.

10
THE STUTTERING
HABIT

TAKING STOCK OF THE INFORMATION I now had, it appeared that stuttering in adults was a physical problem that occurred in response to anticipatory stress. Apparently, it was a sort of psychosomatic disorder.

But what was the somatic or physical component? The Airway Dilation Reflex I saw in young children was absent: no nostril flaring could be noted and none could be felt. All I observed was a fantastic variety of struggling, not only centered about the face but, at various times, throughout all parts of the body. Why this great variety?

I had known for years that one of the things that characterize human beings is the variety of ways in which they learn to cope with adversity. Indeed, one way of looking at different cultures is that they represent different ways in which human beings learn to adapt to adverse natural and man-made conditions. In a sense, a society is the sum total of the coping behaviors of its members.

Was I not observing in all of this variety a sort of testimonial to the diversity of ways in which man responds to and copes with an adverse condition?

Perhaps, but what was this adverse condition? I decided that only one structure had the capability of satisfying the requirement for adversity: the vocal cords. The facts, as described earlier, had pointed consistently to the cords as the likely cause. I decided that the adverse condition was the voluntary tight closure or tensing of the vocal cords just prior to speech, the laryngospasm. This attempt to cope with the Airway Dilation Reflex could be learned quickly and could persist well into adulthood.

With the cords locked together or powerfully tensed the child would not be able to speak, and this would be enough to provoke a variety of struggle behavior designed to release the vocal cords. This behavior, since it led eventually to the production of the desired word, was reinforced and therefore became learned.

As the child grew older, the Airway Dilation Reflex was outgrown. What was left was a chain of these learned stimulus-response reflexes. I concluded, therefore, that stuttering in adults was pure habit.

I now knew why adult stutterers continued to stutter when I brought them to the top of the Empire State Building. All their stuttering was habit. Stress produced the conditioned reflex of vocal cord tension, which, in turn, produced the conditioned reflex of extricatory struggle behavior, the stuttering—a process that can be expressed diagramatically in three stages.

stress → vocal cord tension → stuttering

I now understood why psychotherapy and speech therapy were often ineffective. Neither of these specialties was aware of the existence of the second link in the chain. They were aware only of the two outer links; that is, the therapists heard the patient describe the stresses and observed his struggle behavior. When psychotherapists tried to reduce the stress they would be largely unsuccessful because such stress was sustained by the patient's knowledge that he could not control his blocks at all times. He could not control them because he himself was not aware, first, of all possible sources of stress and, second, of the crucial missing second link in the three-stage process.

The speech therapists, on the other hand, concentrated most often on the observable struggle behavior. Knowing nothing about the locking or tensing of the vocal cords, they were attempting to alter the final phase of a well-established conditioned reflex. The struggle was at the end of a chain; it was automatic and completely programmed. This attempt to prevent stuttering by controlling the struggling in speech now made about as much sense to me as attempting to change the memory of a computer by bending the keys of its teletype output. It was simply too late. The process had to be stopped in the second phase. In other words, the vocal cords had to be

45

prevented from tensing in response to stress. If this could be done, the feedback receptors within the cords would send a different message to the brain, a message that would not have the capability of triggering the conditioned reflex of struggling—and the stutter would abort.

I examined the therapies of the past to see if there were clues in any of them to guide me in proving my theory. I also looked at the enigmas associated with stuttering. The answers abounded. Stutterers often did not stutter when they whispered because they *got set* to whisper by partially opening their vocal cords. This created a new prespeech posture of the vocal cords, a posture that was sensed by the vocal cord feedback receptors and sent to the brain as an entirely different message, a message to which the reflex of stuttering had not been conditioned. And thus the stuttering aborted.

The same was true for singing, for speaking with an assumed southern or foreign accent, for mouthing words silently, and for speaking at a markedly different pitch. The problem with stuttering was a problem in getting set to speak. The patients didn't require speech therapy; what they required was "getting ready to speak" therapy.

The speech therapies of the past often resulted in a change in the pitch of the voice. Sometimes the patient would start his first word an octave higher than usual and then drop down to his normal pitch on the following words. The patients sounded as if they were yodeling, but it did stop their stuttering. Sometimes the patient would be asked to begin in a whisper or sing the first word—all techniques which altered the prespeech posture of the vocal cords.

But these techniques were obtrusive, they called attention to the speech, and the patients simply did not like them. Indeed, many of the techniques used presently are often rejected by patients on the very same grounds.

Furthermore, changing the prespeech posture didn't always work. Patients sometimes still stuttered when whispering or using a different pitch of voice. This was particularly noticeable, the patients reported, when the stress was very high. Perhaps, I thought, under such high stress the patients simply revert to their old habits. Of course, the patients knew nothing about the tensing of the vocal cords and thus were pretty well helpless to do anything constructive to overcome the stuttering block. As a matter of fact, no therapist knew why his technique worked when it did and so obviously could not explain why it often did not work. The technique was more an act of faith than anything else.

11
THE STUTTERER'S
SEVEN BASIC
STRESSES

Since stress is the always-present first link in the three-link chain mentioned previously, I questioned patients about the stresses that provoked their stuttering. I made detailed notes of their descriptions with the purpose of finding common, unifying threads in these observations. Tentative lists of types of stress were prepared and presented to stuttering patients, and critical comments obtained. In this way I developed what I called the stutterer's seven basic stresses.

1. *Situation Stress.* When I asked stutterers in what situation they found speaking most difficult, the most frequent response was, "On the telephone." Over 80 percent of adult stutterers reported some fear of using the phone. I often wondered if the Bell System executives knew that perhaps over a million Americans really dreaded the thought of using this little, essential communication device.

Later I treated a nineteen-year-old man who exemplified this form of stress. He was six foot three and weighed about 220 pounds, and was an exceptional football player. A personable young man, he sat in my office and stuttered moderately in response to my questions.

As is customary in my diagnostic evaluations, I asked him to go to the telephone, call the information operator, and request the telephone number of Macy's Department Store. He refused. I demanded that he do so, saying that this was an essential part of the evaluation. In a split second he was on his knees crying, tugging at my suit jacket, and begging me not to force him to use the telephone. He confessed that he hadn't used it in over ten years and that he had nightmares about it.

A most unusual situation stress was reported by a priest who was terrified of the thought of speaking in the pulpit. His problem had developed in the following manner. He had stuttered as a child, but had outgrown it. After ordination, he assumed a position with a small congregation. In a few years he was given a new post and on his first Sunday entered the church to greet 800 parishioners. The size of the audience overwhelmed him, his vocal cords locked in response to the stress, and the feedback receptors in his cords triggered stuttering responses which had lain dormant for years.

He began to take tranquilizers, but the dosage he required for the drug to be effective created undesirable side effects. He decided to leave the church when his physician told him to stop taking the drugs and he approached his bishop with this decision, saying that his stuttering was apparently a sign of his "unsuitability."

49

The bishop, a practical man, suggested he might try speech therapy before taking so drastic an action.

And so it was that this young priest and I, in the fourth hour of therapy, stood in the pulpit of a local church while he spoke the words of a mass to an empty chapel. Of course, without an audience he didn't stutter, but he was learning a technique I had developed and was practicing it.

We subsequently acquired an audience. First two, then five, then a dozen—while I stood next to him, with my right foot pressed firmly on his left as an ever ready, not so gentle reminder, should he forget to use his new technique.

Parishioners, noticing me occasionally whispering into his ear, thought I was teaching him the techniques for the delivery of the mass. Occasionally they would come up to me after a sermon to compliment me on how well my pupil was doing. If they only knew!

2. *Word or Sound Stress.* Most people who stutter tend to avoid specific words and frequently report that they have difficulty with certain sounds. This form of stress, like almost all forms of stress, is learned. Such learning shows great variability: stutterers can learn to fear any of the sounds, and these fears can change periodically, that is, a person can fear "p" and "t" sounds one year and "s" and "k" sounds the next. Sometimes a person can lose all his fear of specific sounds only to have them return at a later date.

More common are word fears. And almost all adult

stutterers have some of these, very often fearing only a few specific words. I treated a young lawyer who stuttered on only about twenty words and on nothing else. He prepared a list and we concentrated on them. His problem was treated successfully in a few sessions.

I treated another patient who had a problem saying his first name. He had had it legally changed to a name he had always been able to say easily—and then he began to stutter on the new name too. When he saw me he said he was totally unable to say his new name. I encouraged him to try and to continue to make the attempt even though he was having difficulty. I timed it. The block lasted two minutes and thirty-eight seconds—two minutes and thirty-eight seconds of remarkably violent head-thrusting punctuated solely by the occasional need to breathe. His grotesque facial convulsion finally terminated in the speaking of the name David.

Another patient reported invariably lying when asked, "Where did you grow up?" because he could not say Westport. And many patients reported often giving wrong answers in class because they could not say the right ones—and they had to say something. One patient told me he was twenty-eight by saying, "the year after twenty-seven." And many patients bemoaned the fact that they were often required to eat what they did not want to eat in restaurants simply because they were unable to say what they wanted.

Word substitution is, at best, awkward and often frustrating and embarrassing. It is always the result of word or sound stress.

3. *Authority Figure Stress.* Many patients reported having difficulty speaking before individuals best described as authority figures. Such patients had great difficulty talking to the boss or the teacher or when being interviewed.

One patient related that when he was stopped by a policeman for speeding he had to take a sobriety test because he was unable to respond to the officer's questions.

And another patient reported that throughout his school years his questions and answers to teachers were written out and read aloud by fellow students.

4. *The Stress of Uncertainty.* Patients often had difficulty speaking when uncertain about the proper way to behave—for example, in unfamiliar situations such as new neighborhoods or new jobs and meeting new people. This type of stress occurs also when the patient is uncertain about the correct way to pronounce a word.

Nowhere is uncertainty stress more manifest than in the difficulties encountered by stutterers attempting to learn a foreign language. Here the uncertainty is multiplied many times. First an uncertainty about pronunciation, second, one of vocabulary, and third, one of grammar. It is no wonder that some patients reported that they had stuttered on almost every word in the new language.

5. *Physical Stress.* Stutterers sometimes perform more poorly when tired or ill. Indeed, in the nineteenth

century in Europe a school of therapy was devised essentially around the notion that a primary cause of stuttering was a lack of sleep. And so patients were often required to sleep as many as fourteen hours a day as a treatment.

Some early therapists believed that only a certain part of the body—usually the tongue—was tired, and various devices were constructed to hold up the "tired" tongue. Generally made of gold or ivory, and worn in the mouth, such devices functioned essentially as distractions and, as such, temporarily stopped the stuttering. But after a few days, at most, the stuttering returned with as much intensity as ever.

6. *External Stress.* This form of stress can also be called "bad news." It is the stress of discovering that you have just been fired or that a relative has a terminal illness or that your car has been stolen. Patients reported that external stress figured prominently in their difficulty.

I treated a patient who responded beautifully to my techniques and after a few days of intensive therapy was symptom-free in virtually all situations. He left for his home in Ohio confident of his new skills and equally certain that the continuation of his program at home would strengthen these new habits and establish them permanently.

When he returned, however, he discovered that his house had been burglarized and burned. The external stress was so great that it took him fully six weeks to regain his ability to control his stuttering.

53

I have seen patients operating in the pressure cooker of the advertising world who, while fluent in most situations after treatment, cannot cope with the external stress of clients continuously contemplating agency changes.

7. *Speed Stress.* Probably the most important of all the stresses is speed stress. Speed stress is undoubtedly reponsible for the onset of most stuttering in children. It is the product of speaking too rapidly.

Almost all patients were found to suffer from this in some degree. For very young children, speed stress was often the only form of stress they experienced. When they spoke slowly, they became fluent. Adults, on the other hand, were under other forms of stress, and thus slow speaking did not result in immediate fluency for most.

As a matter of fact, most adults were not aware of speaking too rapidly. Indeed, when I measured the average number of words they spoke per minute, when fluent, it was well within normal limits; it was not a question of the average number of words per minute but rather of how quickly they spoke the first word in each sentence; that is, how quickly they started to speak.

When this was measured, they were found to be as much as four times faster than average. In other words, stutterers tend to attack their words, instead of beginning speech in a slow and leisurely manner.

One patient who invariably stuttered on the first word of each sentence indicated that the reason he spoke his first word so quickly was that he "wanted to get away from the scene of the crime as quickly as possible." What he did not realize, of course, was that this desire was resulting in speed stress and thereby helping to contribute to the very block he was seeking to escape.

12
BASELINE
STRESS

THERE IS YET ANOTHER stress to consider—separately, as it is quite distinct from the seven basic stresses. I call it the baseline stress. It is defined as the amount of tension in the muscles of the body at any one moment. It is the result of a number of influences, many of which are subconscious. For example, we are all aware of the experience of going into a room and finding ourselves uncomfortable and tense without knowing why. Something in the room, beneath our level of consciousness, is provoking a stress response. Some mornings we wake up with stress, that is, with tension, and on other mornings with a sense of profound relaxation.

The vocal cords are extremely sensitive indicators of baseline stress. When the baseline stress is high the vocal cords show a high level of tension. When any of the other stresses are present, the tension in the vocal cords produced by these stresses is added to that caused by the already high baseline stress and the feedback receptors in the vocal cords trigger the stuttering reflex. It is during these times of high baseline stress that patients and the parents of young patients report having "a difficult time."

On the other hand, if the baseline stress is low, the addition of any one of the other stresses may not provoke enough tension in the cords to elicit the reflex of stuttering, and the patient then reports he is having "an easy time."

Thus, the patient seeking a solution to his problem may go to a psychiatrist who eventually succeeds in lowering the patient's baseline stress. The patient then experiences "improvement."

But if he subsequently encounters a multiple-stress situation, his vocal cords may lock and the result will be the inevitable block. When the block does occur, he feels helpless, and this may result in an increased baseline stress, and the patient has then "relapsed." So it's back to the psychiatrist for another year or two.

Baseline stress fluctuates widely in young children, accounting for the alternating periods of fluency and nonfluency reported by parents. Many children come to my office during one of their fluent periods. Their parents assure me that their children do stutter and sometimes violently, and in a sense they apologize for their child's fluent performance. They almost invariably say that they are unable to account for such fluctuations and they experience much reduction of guilt when I explain baseline stress to them and indicate that the fluency fluctuation in young children is often largely the result of something as uncontrollable as periodic fluctuations in

57

the chemistry of the nerve cells making up the human brain.

A marked increase in baseline stress was responsible for the reemergence of stuttering in a young man in his mid twenties after a period of some eighteen years of relative fluency. It appears that about a year prior to my seeing him he had received some bad news, that is, an external stress. He had been told that his father was very ill, perhaps terminally, and this information and the constant worrying it provoked resulted in an elevation of his baseline stress.

When I saw him he was stuttering mostly on vowels. His struggles were minimal in severity but unmistakable. Because he had been fluent for such a long period of time, I was able to treat him successfully in five one-hour sessions.

13
A COMBINATION
OF
STRESSES

SIMULTANEOUS, MULTIPLE STRESSES are common-place; we rarely function in single-stress environments. I very often tell patients to imagine the following situation: "You have had a sleepless night and are not feeling well. Your boss, out of town on a business trip, calls you and asks you to quickly find the name of a chemical that he needs desperately for a specific purpose (you know the name of the chemical—it begins with a sound you cannot produce and also it is so long you are not certain about its pronunciation) and if you don't find that name quickly he threatens to fire you." Let's analyze this improbable situation.

The "not feeling well" is physical stress. The "boss" is authority figure stress. The telephone is situation stress. The "hurry up" is speed stress. The feared sound falls within word and sound stress. The uncertainty of pronunciation falls in the category of uncertainty stress. And the threat of being "fired" is obviously external stress. Under these conditions it would not be surprising to find the patient unable to say anything at all.

The point of this story is that stress can be multiple and additive and that the greater the stress, the tighter the lockup of the vocal cords.

When a patient is alone and speaking to himself out loud he is under what I call a "minimal stress condition." In such a condition there is no tension on the vocal cords and therefore no stuttering. This is true even though the baseline stress may be high.

It is easy to see, then, why most stutterers report no difficulty speaking to animals or young children; the stress is so low in these conditions that there is not enough tension in the vocal cords to trigger the block.

14
THE SELF-STRESSER

A FINAL ASPECT of the subject of stress has to do with a type of individual whom I call the "self-stresser." The self-stresser is a person who overreacts to his stuttering —who views the occurrence of a block as an event of devastating proportion. This individual continuously re-elevates his baseline stress; he lacks the capability for tranquil response to nonfluency.

Among the first patients I treated was a fifty-three-year-old anesthesiologist who had stuttered violently all his life. (There are only three specialties in medicine within which stutterers usually can comfortably practice: anesthesiology, radiology, and pathology.)

As an anesthesiologist, he immediately understood the concept of the Airway Dilation Reflex and within an hour of treatment was symptom-free. We spent several days together reinforcing his new habits and not once during that time did he stutter. He returned to his position at an Upper New York State hospital and remained totally symptom-free for a period of almost three months. During this time he used the telephone daily, gave lectures to students and colleagues, and participated in all routine speaking situations.

One day, however, he encountered an unexpected four-stress speaking situation, his larynx went into spasm, and he stuttered. He reached me at eleven that evening and opened his conversation with the statement, "The edifice is crumbling." His baseline stress had risen to the point where his stuttering had returned in just a few hours to its pretherapy levels.

I was incredulous. How could a man who had been fluent for three months suddenly revert so completely? The answer lay in the perfection of his speech. Having been totally fluent for over twelve weeks, he had developed an entirely unrealistic attitude about his speech, a sort of false confidence. And when the first block did occur, as it must inevitably, he responded irrationally and raised his baseline stress to a level that resulted in virtually continuous stuttering. While he was in this tense state, each block served to propel his baseline higher in what I was later to recognize as a classic self-stressing mode. Fully two months elapsed before this man was able to regain his composure and use the techniques he had been taught. During that time he was given instructions designed to temper his tendency toward self-defeating responses. When he regained fluency he did it with the wisdom gleaned from this experience and so has remained symptom-free.

15
HAIR-PULLING
AND
PENCIL-TOSSING

OTHER FEATURES ASSOCIATED with stuttering remained enigmatic. For example, how was one to evaluate the young child who pulled a hair out of her head to release herself from a block, or the man who could speak only by timing the onset of his sentences to the act of throwing a pencil into the air? How and why did these actions work? How did they fit into the three-link chain (stress—vocal cord tension—stuttering)?

The answer became clear when I considered the subject of distraction.

Many stutterers asserted that if they could do something to distract their attention their stuttering would abate. For example, when one patient felt a block coming he would put his hand in his pocket and start to pinch his thigh. The pain would distract his attention away from his anticipatory stress and he would not stutter. Thus, for this patient, thigh-pinching served as a covert but socially acceptable anticipatory coping behavior designed to deal with stress.

Another patient reported biting the inside of his

cheek while in a block as a means of releasing himself from it. As in the case of the child who pulled a hair from her head, the pain of the activity distracted the attention of the brain away from the feedback signals from the tensed cords, thus aborting the stuttering.

The difference between the cheek biter and the hair puller lay in the issue of social acceptability. The former was a socially acceptable covert behavior; the latter a socially unacceptable overt one.

I discussed the subject of distraction with a colleague, an experimental psychologist whose broad knowledge of the literature on the relationship between brain and behavior was to be of much help to me in developing my ideas. As we sat at lunch one day, he described an interesting experiment.

Apparently one can locate an area on the outer surface of the cat's brain which responds to sound impulses coming up from the animal's ears. That is, a clicking noise near a cat's ear will produce increased electrical activity in the portion of the cat's brain responsible for hearing sound.

The experimenters, through surgery, implanted a minute wire in this portion of the brain and fed the other end of it out through the skull to a sensitive recording instrument. An electronic clicker introduced into the cat's environment made a continuous series of sharp, poplike sounds. The instruments recorded discrete electrical impulses from the cat's brain which corresponded to each sound. At this point a small mouse was introduced into the cage. As soon as the cat saw the mouse, the sound signals from the cat's brain ceased, even though the popping sound continued.

The visual presence of the mouse had distracted the cat. Here was evidence of the brain's ability to suppress information coming from one area of sensation in order to focus more intently upon information coming from another. The brain had shifted its attention, and here was the direct physical evidence to prove it.

Thus what we were seeing in the distraction devices employed by stuttering patients was a clear-cut expression of the ability of the brain to focus its attention selectively from one mental point of view to another. Unfortunately, the distraction often had to be intense and so was usually either painful or bizarre. If the distraction was mild, it might lose its distracting capabilities quickly and the stuttering would then reappear.

Many therapies in the past have made use of distraction devices. In the eighteenth century in Europe, for example, itinerant "doctors" offered a variety of magical cures for stuttering. Sometimes the cure was a wad of cotton supposedly treated with a magical fluid that would cure stuttering. The patient would take a piece of this cotton, roll it into a ball about the size of a grape, and place it under his tongue and then speak. The presence of a large mass under the tongue during speech served as a distraction and the stuttering ceased. The patient was instructed to replace the cotton every few hours with a fresh one, since the "fluid would lose its potency after a while." As soon as the distraction of speaking with cotton under the tongue wore off, and this sometimes took a day or a week, the stuttering returned. By that time, however, the "doctor" was out of town.

The figure below shows another distraction device employed in the treatment of stuttering. Basically an or-

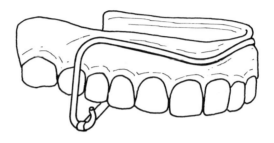

thodontic appliance fitted into the upper jaw, the Freed Stammercheck interfered with normal speech production and therefore served in a distracting capacity:

It has been said that well over fifty patents have been issued by the United States Patent Office for essentially distraction devices designed to treat stuttering. There has been no lack of interest.

A description of the devices designed to control stuttering, written by a Mr. Potter in 1882, serves to indicate the extent to which a stutterer will go to overcome his affliction:

> They cost $35, are patented and consist of three articles, (1) a coin-silver instrument in the form of a small flattened bedpan worn in the mouth with the handle projecting between the lips, for the purpose of giving access to air and egress to the breath in labial stuttering; (2) a small gold tube to

be attached by a rubber band to one of the teeth for the relief of the dental form of stuttering; (3) a larynx compressor, capable of increasing pressure by tightening up a screw and a buckle, attached to a band for the neck to be worn by those who have difficulty in enunciating the gutterals. As nearly every serious case presents all the forms mentioned, the simultaneous use of the three appliances would be necessary in order to be prepared for any emergency.

Even today patients come to my office wearing what appears to be a hearing aid behind their ear but which, in reality, is an electronic metronome clicking at a prescribed rate. The purpose of the metronome presumably is to give them a rhythm to which they can time their syllables. This device is, in part, a distraction, but since it is very often set at a slow speed, its effect is also to slow the speech and thereby reduce speed stress.

Other patients report learning to make specific movements with their hands and arms as a distracting prelude to speech. These movements are usually rhythmical and form a pattern, and speech can begin only when a certain feature of the pattern is achieved. For example, a speech therapist who is also a stutterer once told me that he was taught to swing his right arm, making a figure eight in the air, and that he could begin to speak only when the lines crossed. He reported that this worked for a short while but that he gave it up when it ceased to distract and started to become nothing more than another bizarre accompaniment to his stuttering.

Perhaps the most interesting distraction of all was reported to me by a patient who at an earlier stage in his life had moved from New Jersey to California, changed his name, his manner of speech, and as much as possible all features of his prior existence—his style of clothing, his haircut, his mode of living, even his habits of thought. He distracted himself into believing he was someone else, feeling that if he was successful at this he would be "reborn" a fluent person. And it worked for a while, until one day, in a restaurant, he met someone from his former "life." Caught off guard, he reverted to his old manner of responding, his cords locked, and he stuttered. This so unnerved him that his baseline stress rose considerably and his old habits returned. The ultimate distraction had failed.

16
THE FOUR TYPES
OF
STUTTERING

WITH THIS BACKGROUND of understanding, I began to study the variety of struggle in the adult stutterers I saw. Although there were many types of struggle, I was able to decipher four major categories.

Type I

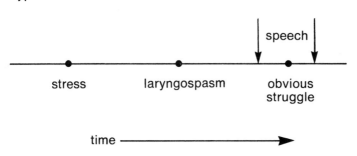

A diagram of the first category, Type I, shows the normal type of stuttering. The horizontal line indicates time moving from left to right. The three dots on the line indicate the three links of stuttering, that is, from stress to laryngospasm to stuttering. So we see in this diagram that the onset of stress leads to the laryngospasm which shortly precedes the struggles *in* speech.

The second category is indicated by the Type II diagram. Again stress leads to the laryngospasm which

Type II

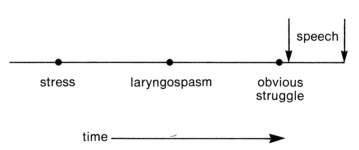

provokes a struggle, though in this instance it is not part of speech but precedes it. The struggling may be violent but the stutterer has elected to delay his speech until after the struggle—so his speech is always fluent.

I treated several patients with this type of stuttering. The patient mentioned earlier, whose speech was preceded by violent backward thrusts of his head, was an example. This man never struggled with any speech sound; rather, the struggling always occurred before the beginning of speech.

In Type III stuttering the stress also provokes the laryngospasm, but the patient with this form of the disorder has elected not to struggle but rather to pause

Type III

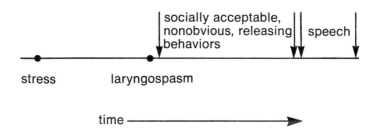

and wait until the laryngospasm releases. This may be accomplished by several means: he may distract himself in some appropriate manner, he may passively wait for his stress to drop, he may quietly inhale to open his vocal cords, or he may swallow to achieve the same end. One patient I treated would cough gently during such pauses to blow his vocal cords apart.

Finally, the last diagram shows Type IV stuttering, in which the three-link chain is aborted before it starts. The stutterer distracts himself or uses an avoidance behavior when his scanner informs him of the presence of "trouble ahead."

Type I stuttering is the "typical" form, seen most often in stutterers. The struggles are associated with speech and with certain sounds. Type II stuttering, though less frequent, is also recognized as stuttering even though the speech is unimpaired. Type III and Type IV stuttering are socially acceptable; they are not recog-

71

Type IV

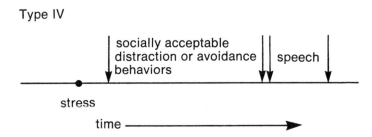

nized as forms of stuttering. Stutterers in these two categories rarely seek professional help even though these
types of the disorder often take a considerable personal
emotional toll.

As I examined more and more adult stutterers, I was
to discover mixtures of each of these four types. For
example, a patient might struggle with the pronunciation
of his name, substitute one word for another while describing his occupation, and cough to release his laryngospasm before describing an experience. I was to discover
that a mixture of types within patients was the rule
rather than the exception. There were, of course, "pure"
types, and clinicians would see them on occasion. They
were mostly Type I and Type II. Types III and IV were
rarely seen, not because they did not exist in substantial
numbers, but rather because, as I have mentioned, they
did not seek assistance.

17
COMMON
STRUGGLES

I NOW LOOKED DIRECTLY at the struggles. They were of a great variety. Sometimes a patient would lock his vocal cords very tightly and show no displacement of struggle to any other structure. He would report that he used to struggle openly, but had learned to suppress these struggles and, in so doing, considered that he had improved. But now he was stuck, literally, having focused all his struggle upon the vocal cords. What he did not realize was that he simply had shifted from Type I stuttering to Type III.

Type I stuttering behaviors can be considered as various ways in which human beings can learn to struggle in speech to release a laryngospasm. So, for example, a person might press his lips together forcefully to produce a "p" sound only to find them locked there and unable to proceed. The tendency to open the lips is accomplished in English "p" sounds only when the vocal cords are open. If the vocal cords are in a locked position, opening of the lips will produce no sound and thus the lips, through conditioning, stay firmly together until the lockup is removed.

This same condition applies for a variety of speech sounds. The patient believes his stuttering is located in his mouth because he can sense the struggling taking place there. But he never asks himself the question, struggling against what? The answer, of course, is the laryngospasm.

Sometimes a patient will repeat a sound rather than hold it in a fixed position. Thus a patient might repeat the "p" sound several times in an effort to proceed with the rest of the word. This type of repetition is what some therapists call clonic stuttering, whereas locking the lips together in a fixed position for "p" production, as in the previous example, is called tonic stuttering. Elaborate theories have been developed to account for these two forms of stuttering, but the explanation is really quite simple.

Several years ago, while riding on the Penn Central train between New York and Philadelphia, I had occasion to observe an interesting spectacle. Sitting at one end of the car, I could see passengers coming into the car from the one ahead. In order to enter they had to push a horizontal bar labeled "Push" to open the door. What these people did not know was that the bar was inoperative and when the bar was pushed the door would not budge. There were two sorts of reactions to this unexpected impediment in the forward progress of my cotravelers. One group, finding the "Push" bar unresponsive would, with added force, push rapidly and repeatedly until it opened, while the other group would simply lean heavily against it and push continuously until it opened. Here, then, was clonic and tonic pushing. These were simply two ways in which human beings react to the sudden, unexpected, and complete arrestation of an ongoing movement pattern.

I observed one passenger come into the car a second time. As he approached the door, he lifted his foot and with a mighty kick slammed the push bar so that the door flew open. Here was the analogy for a "severe" stutterer if I ever saw one.

18
CHURCHILL'S LONG "M" AND OTHER STARTERS

I BEGAN TO OBSERVE a set of mannerisms called starters, used by many stutterers to prevent their vocal cords from locking. The function of a starter is to keep the vocal cords vibrating just prior to the act of speaking. With the cords engaged in such activity, they cannot go into spasm—and when there is no spasm, of course, there is no stuttering. Thus, for example, one often hears the sound "uh" preceding feared words; in this case, if the patient is asked to leave this sound out he stutters. Sometimes, however, a patient begins to stutter on his starter; to cope with his, he may add another word or sound as a new starter to enable him to go on to produce his old one so that he can proceed to say the word he intends to say. Sometimes a string of starters can be as long as four or five words. Usually they are in some reasonably socially acceptable form. For example, "uh lemme see uh" may appear before almost every sentence.

One of the most famous starters of all time was the one developed by Winston Churchill to conquer his stuttering in adolescence. He later turned this starter into a well-known personal oratorical style. What he did was to place a long "m" at the beginning of some of his sentences. Many of us remember his style: "Mmmmmm-mmmEngland will never surrender." In this case, the "m," of course, kept his vocal cords vibrating and enabled him to proceed with his sentences without a laryngospasm.

While Winston Churchill's starter was a socially acceptable coping behavior, others chosen by patients are often not so successful. Take, for example, one of my patients who would respond to his anticipated difficulty with a word by repeating the word that went before it. If he still felt he would stutter, he would repeat the prior word once again. Sometimes he would say the prior word as many as fifteen or twenty times. And if that failed, he would start repeating the prior two words, perhaps as many as five or six times. These repetitions were effortless; he had no difficulty saying these words—it was the word that was not spoken, the word that was to come next with which he had difficulty. Ironically, most of his listeners knew that he was a stutterer because they heard all these examples of "stuttering." Little did they realize that they never heard him stutter once but were simply listening to a socially unacceptable set of anticipatory coping behaviors.

Thus, I discovered that repetitions did not always constitute stuttering and that starters were an extremely pervasive device used for aborting the stuttering block.

19
THE READINESS
IS ALL

MANY PATIENTS STUTTERED only at the beginning of
sentences, as if the act of getting set to speak was the
factor provoking the laryngospasm. Other patients,
however, stuttered in the middle of sentences; some even
stuttered on every word. How could one account for
this? Didn't the words at the beginning of sentences serve
as "starters," and, if so, wouldn't they successfully prevent stuttering on a word in the middle of a sentence? It
appeared that this was true in a large percentage of patients, particularly those who had no word or sound
stress. But if a patient did have a substantial amount of
word or sound stress, he would often stop momentarily
just before the word, thereby enabling himself to get set
to say the word; while getting set he would tense his
vocal cords, and then he would stutter. When I forced
patients not to stop before their feared words, the preceding word then functioned as a starter and the stuttering aborted.

Thus, I came to the conclusion that whenever a patient stutters he does so because he has stopped and is

having trouble getting started. I now understood one of the reasons why stuttering was eliminated during singing —the continuous melodic line provided scant opportunity for a pause within which a laryngospasm might occur.

I remembered a sentence from a soliloquy by Hamlet: "The readiness is all." Stutterers were stutterers because their readiness to speak was all wrong.

It is the way stutterers get set to speak that I realized I had to concentrate on in my search for an effective technique for preventing stuttering.

PART II
The Treatment

20
DEVELOPING
AIRFLOW
THERAPY

I NOW TURNED to the task of developing a therapy. The problem was to alter the prespeech postures of the vocal cords in a way that would not be detectable by listeners. Patients simply did not care to go about singing, whispering, mouthing their words silently, or speaking in breathy voices. They wanted something that sounded normal, and I couldn't say I blamed them.

In the final stages of the development of my theory of stuttering, I interviewed a number of persons who had stuttered badly as children but who had later outgrown it. My purpose was to examine their speech for clues to the successful coping behaviors they had developed in overcoming their problem.

My interviews revealed some patients speaking a bit more slowly than usual, though this did not seem particularly remarkable. On the other hand, I found a substantial number exhibiting what appeared to be tiny airflows in their speech: I could detect a small amount of air coming from their mouths just before they spoke. It was as if they spoke with a tiny sigh before each of their sentences.

The more I thought about this, the more intrigued I became. Why these airflows? What function did they serve? I never heard them in the speech of stutterers, nor in the speech of normal speakers with no history of stuttering. Why, then, in this group?

I remember sitting in my office with my pipe in my mouth, mimicking these flows, watching the smoke come out prior to each sentence. And then it hit me. The answer was in the flow. The flow was being used to ensure an opening of the vocal cords prior to speaking. The flow was passive, never pushed, and its sighlike quality kept the cords apart and relaxed.

I could now explain the bizarre behavior of a patient who had come to me several years earlier and stated that he never stuttered when he smoked. When I asked him to demonstrate, he lit a cigarette, inhaled, let out some of the smoke, and began to speak. The stuttering disappeared.

When I asked him why he thought it helped him, he said that smoking relaxed him. I had passed it off as a well-learned distraction device. Little did I suspect at that time that the answer to the problem was to be seen in the smoke being blown past my face.

I now began to experiment with an airflow technique. I started by asking a stutterer to produce a long, audible, and relaxed sigh. I then asked him to sigh once again, and when halfway through it, to say a one-syllable word. The stuttering aborted immediately. I increased the number of one-syllable words spoken on a breath. Again, there was no stuttering.

I was amazed. It all seemed too simple. Was I being taken in by another distraction device? Was I, albeit in sophisticated fashion, just repeating what hundreds had attempted before me?

But, day after day, the patient's speech continued to be fluent. My spirits began to rise. I kept wondering how long before the inevitable relapse, but it did not occur, and I decided to proceed to the next step. I asked the patient to make the flow totally inaudible. He did this immediately, saying he had practiced this at home since he did not care to go about sounding "like a breathy pervert." His speech was now totally acceptable. His voice quality was normal, the flow was undetectable, and, of course, he was not stuttering.

Here, I thought, was a treatment that represented the essence of simplicity. It focused specifically upon what the theory postulated as the major cause of stuttering. The passive airflow kept the vocal cords open and relaxed prior to speech and thus the brain was deprived of the feedback signals necessary to trigger the conditioned reflex of stuttering.

21
MISUSES
OF
AIRFLOW

I was soon to discover, however, that for certain patients, the immediacy of the result belied a subsequent period of difficulty. Although they used the airflow continuously, they still stuttered at times. What was wrong?

I paid careful attention to these occurrences as they appeared in the tape recordings several patients had made for me. Later, when listening to their tapes and examining subtle aspects of the flows, I was able to uncover five characteristics which seemed to provoke the reappearance of stuttering. I called them misuses of air flow, and all patients were subsequently given explicit instructions to alert them to these pitfalls and enable them to avoid them.

1. *Pushing the Flow.* Under conditions of stress, patients tended to push the flow, which frequently led to a laryngospasm and a subsequent stutter.

Patients were warned that the flow had to be absolutely passive; that they were to inhale, relax, and let the flow come out without effort; then while the air was flowing in this manner, they were to begin to speak. They were told that a pushed flow would sooner or later be interpreted by the brain as an "h." The brain would then "think" that all sentences began with "h" and hence the patient might begin to stutter on it. Pushing the flow was never to be allowed.

2. *A Failure of Transition.* Another source of trouble was the lack of a smooth flow into the first sounds the patients wished to say. The flow stopped short, with a slight pause between the end of the flow and the beginning of the sound. This pause provided all the time necessary for the occurrence of a laryngospasm.

To avoid stuttering the patient must not interrupt the passive flow of the air that leads directly into speech. This is relatively simple to do for almost all the sounds, the exceptions being the explosive sounds (p, t, k, b, d, g)—and for these the airflow must be as close to the sound as possible.

3. *A Failure of Intent.* Patients often are so preoccupied with the upcoming sound that their mouths are formed into position for that sound at the beginning of the airflow. Thus, the flow of air is affected by the anticipated sound, and one of the effects can be a tensing of the vocal cords, a tensing that leads to laryngospasm.

Patients were instructed that the primary intent must always be the flow, and that when the air was flowing, then and only then were they to shift their intent and begin to speak. Failure of intent was an important

87

problem which appeared most often under stressful conditions.

4. *Holding the Flow*. One patient, in an effort to time the flows properly, would inhale and hold the air by closing his vocal cords, and then start the airflow at the appropriate time by releasing his cords. If he attempted to do this under conditions of stress, the hold would be transformed into a locking of his vocal cords and he would stutter.

Patients were instructed never to hold the flow but rather to keep the air in constant movement, that is, to inhale smoothly and then just as smoothly reverse the flow and exhale; there was never to be a stoppage of flow.

5. *Omitting the Flow*. This usually occurs because of distraction and rarely because of stress, and becomes less and less of a problem as the patient continues to practice and gets into what I call a "flow groove." Omitting the flow, while quite common at the very beginning of therapy, is relatively rare after the first week.

22
A PRESCRIPTION
FOR
FLUENCY

MY PATIENTS WERE now responding well. The flow technique, when practiced properly, brought substantial improvement. But occasionally stuttering blocks occurred: despite the use of seemingly perfect airflows, some patients still stuttered at times.

Reexamining these patients, I would, for example, hear a young man use the flow technique perfectly into a "t" and then start to struggle. Why did this patient suddenly go into laryngospasm? There had to be some form of stress present. I tape-recorded a collection of some fifty instances of these unexplainable blocks and played them over and over.

I was listening to them at home one evening, wondering if I would ever find a solution, when my wife entered the den commenting, "You know, those people speak awfully fast." And then I realized the obvious fact —they were speed-stressing themselves.

It turned out that if a patient was "hung up" on a sound, though properly using the flow technique into it, it would be a virtual certainty that the syllable of which that sound was the initial component would be spoken extremely rapidly. Thus when I forced patients to pronounce the first syllable after each flow slowly, the stuttering aborted completely.

The explanation was that the first syllable was produced rapidly because the speaker's intent to say it rapidly preceded the syllable and coincided in time with the flow, thus affecting it. The speed stress caused the vocal cords to tense during the flow, and as the sound was produced, the tension progressed to the state of laryngospasm, and the stuttering block occurred. In a sense, it was a form of failure of intent, but in this instance it was a failure of the intent to say the first syllable slowly.

I treated a patient who exemplified this condition. An executive at one of the country's largest commercial banks, he stuttered at the beginning of virtually every sentence. He was a Type II stutterer; that is, all of his struggle preceded the onset of the first sound. Listening to him over the phone, all one ever heard were slight pauses before each sentence—but watching him was quite another matter. The fierce silent struggles which preceded each sentence were awesome. It was no wonder he was housed in a small, out-of-the-way office—out of the sight of everyone.

When I evaluated his problem I discovered two things. First, he did indeed stutter only at the beginnings of sentences. And, second, the first words of each sentence were spoken approximately three and a half times faster than normal.

It turned out that this man was a pure speed stresser. He had none of the other stresses. When I taught him to slow the first syllable of each sentence, his stuttering aborted immediately. Airflow was not necessary since the tensing of the cords was being provoked only by speed stress. I treated this man successfully in a few sessions and his speech has remained fluent.

I now realized that if a patient adhered to the passive flow technique and slowed the first syllable after the flow he could not stutter even if he wanted to. I began to inform patients of this very important fact. I proposed that if they obeyed this twofold rule, they would be physiologically unable to stutter. I arranged multiple-stress speaking situations so that each patient could see firsthand that this dictum was inevitably true. The effect of the patient's successful performance in these situations was powerful and obvious. In addition, no one had ever told him anything quite as simple yet startlingly dogmatic. Here, for the first time, was a specific and clear-cut prescription for fluency. Patients invariably responded to this startling discovery by experiencing a sharp drop in their baseline stress.

23
STARTING
INTENSIVE THERAPY

ALTHOUGH I WAS TREATING patients now with some measure of success, I discovered that seeing a patient for an hour once or twice a week left too great an opportunity for undesirable regression between sessions. I knew that many therapies for stuttering in the past had used intensive treatment techniques and I decided to try one as well. The results turned out to be so remarkably superior that I have adhered to this technique ever since.

In the first phase of treatment adult patients are seen eight hours a day for five consecutive days. In this phase the patient is literally blitzed by both information and practice. He is given the details of how stuttering begins, instructed in the seven basic stresses, told about the misuses of airflow that can occur, and provided with some knowledge of the anatomy and physiology of the speaking mechanism, as well as of the principles of learning. And after being shown the airflow technique, he is given an opportunity to use it in virtually every stress condition imaginable.

92

Typically, at the end of the week, patients are symptom-free in virtually all situations. The results with approximately 185 patients were that 89 percent of them were completely symptom-free in all situations within the week.

But one week of intensive therapy is not enough to establish a totally new pattern of behavior, and the results just mentioned must be reinforced by a second phase of therapy—the phase of habit reinforcement. Though symptom-free after the first week, the patient still has 98 percent of the work ahead of him. He possesses all the relevant information, but the new habit has virtually no strength and the old habit (the laryngospasm), which has been practiced literally millions of times, is still incredibly strong.

Accordingly, the patient must practice one hour daily for a year. The one hour is divided into four 15-minute sessions. One minute of each of these sessions is recorded on tape, and the patient sends to me each week a cassette with twenty-eight of the one-minute taped segments for evaluation. Each tape is heard, my comments are recorded on it, together with the next week's assignment, and the cassette is then sent back to the patient. In this manner the patient is monitored on a weekly basis to make sure that he does not develop undesirable habits, that motivational levels are kept high, and that the strength of the habit is built on a formal and systematic basis.

This procedure, which has proven to be highly successful, enables me to continue treatment, after the first week of therapy, with patients living at a considerable distance from my office. Long-term follow-up indicates that 83 percent of my patients have remained symptom-free after one year.

24
KEYS
TO PREVENTING
RELAPSE

In the course of the intensive phase of therapy it soon became apparent that the achievement of quick fluency was not without its penalty. The immediacy and pervasiveness of the fluency often caused an extremely rapid drop in the patient's baseline stress. The patient acquired great confidence that sometimes bordered on cockiness. The stage was now set for disregarding the airflow technique.

Since the baseline stress had dropped, patients found themselves not stuttering even though they failed to use the flow. Such patients were forcefully reprimanded and told that if they did not use the flow before every sentence I would give them a written guarantee that they would surely stutter again. To emphasize this point, I would arrange to place the patient in a multiple-stress situation that would precipitate a laryngospasm and a stutter. In this way the patient was brought quickly back to reality and shown that the airflow was to be a permanent accompaniment to the act of speaking and not something that might be used only when needed. Unless the flow of air was automatic and habitual it would ultimately fail in high-stress situations.

I had learned my lesson from the anesthesiologist. I was not going to permit any patient to build false confidence in himself. The patients had to realize that they had learned to stutter and that they would have to "learn their way out of the problem." The elimination of stuttering was not a passive act. It required application, motivation, and practice. I often told patients: "Getting you fluent is absolutely no challenge at all. Keeping you fluent is the name of the game." It is a game that most patients, once suddenly freed from the albatross around their necks, were very willing to play.

During this period of therapy evolution I often reread descriptions of the therapies of the past. One of the things that struck me about prior attempts to treat stuttering was that patients were always called upon to learn techniques by rote.

They were told to talk slowly, or to relax, or to control their blocks by easing out of them, or to swing their arms, or to speak to the rhythm of a metronome—but never why. The attitude was that understanding either bore no relation to the therapy or was of no importance. Of course, many clinicians had no understanding of why certain therapies did or did not work but were, themselves, rote practitioners.

This was entirely unsatisfactory. It accounted for why patients and therapists often got nowhere and why the occasional initial success often disintegrated. I recognized that I had to make understanding the foundation of my therapy. I realized that if the patient viewed stuttering as an enigmatic affliction, he would be manipulated and victimized by it. Instead, the patient had to be shown that his stuttering was pure habit, that it represented an orderly chain of stimulus-response learning, and that the struggling was at the end of the chain and therefore could not be the focus of attention for therapy.

Many times during the course of the intensive first phase I had to refresh patients' memories that we were concerned exclusively with the way they got set to speak. They were made to visualize and sense the state of tension within their vocal cords before they spoke, to recognize that if they did stutter they had simply allowed themselves to go into laryngospasm. As the occurrence of a stuttering block could always be explained in a logical manner, the patients were encouraged to find the reason in each instance. Had they misused the airflow? Did they fail to slow the first syllable following the flow? Were they subjected to a multiple-stress situation? These were some of the questions that patients were trained to ask and answer for themselves.

Once the patient saw he was capable of understanding what he was doing wrong, or what factors were present to contribute to the block, stuttering lost its mystery. And when the mystery was taken from it, former emotional responses were replaced by coolly analytical ones, the baseline stress was kept from rising, and the occurrence of a relapse was made far more remote.

25
SEVERE
STUTTERING

MOST OF MY COLLEAGUES generally identify a severe stutterer as one who struggles severely and often. From my point of view, however, this emphasis on overt struggle is misplaced. Violent, overt struggling is simply an individual response to the occurrence of a laryngospasm. It represents a socially unacceptable coping behavior.

What I consider to be severe stuttering has nothing at all to do with the magnitude of the viewable struggle, but is associated with the intensity of the patient's stress level and the firmness and frequency of the laryngospasm. In my experience, severe stutterers constitute no more than about 12 percent of the patients.

To understand the role of stress in severe stuttering, it is important to realize that human beings react differently to an unexpected impediment in the progression of speech. Part of this different way of reacting is learned and part is inherited. I call people who react excessively to speech difficulties "Chihuahuas." In contrast to the Chihuahua, the toy poodle scurries about the feet of human beings, brazenly moving about with no apparent fear. But the Chihuahua is always fearful—shaking, quivering, almost as if it expected each moment to be its last. When a stutterer reacts like a Chihuahua with exaggerated stress responses, it may be exceedingly difficult to help him.

I have treated patients far too fearful even to breathe quietly in response to my request to do so. I have seen patients go into a rigid position of panic, automatically lock their vocal cords, and remain totally unresponsive to any physical prodding (even a painful one) until their moment of panic had run its course. One patient with very high word stress told me that as he spoke he would visualize a conveyor belt carrying the words toward him. He would scan the belt for any approaching feared word, which he saw as engraved on a tombstone. As the tombstone bearing the feared word approached, he could feel his heartbeat accelerate. He would experience a progressive tightening in his chest and throat. And when the stone got very close, his mind would go blank and he would be trapped in a special vise of panic—a panic so great that he would stutter even if he were alone and spoke out loud to himself.

Later I was to ask patients routinely if they ever stuttered when they spoke aloud to themselves. If the response was positive, the prognosis for the patient was less than ideal.

One patient reported extremely high word stress for saying his name. When someone introduced himself to him, he could never hear the name of the person to whom he was being introduced because of his panic in the knowledge that he would soon have to say his own name. Only later would the patient learn the names of those to whom he had previously been introduced.

Patients with such a great degree of stress very often did not possess the requisite presence of mind required for airflow use. My technique, in these circumstances, was inadequate and so I turned to other clinical specialties for assistance. I sent my patients for hypnosis, transcendental meditation, psychiatry (and the use of tranquilizers), and behavior modification—all with limited success. The most promising of these has been behavior modification. And this approach may hold the solution to the problem of the extremely high-stress patient.

The second component in my definition of severity is the frequency and firmness of the laryngospasm. In most patients stuttering appeared only at the beginning of sentences and the incidence of their stuttering was relatively low; others stuttered on several words in each sentence. In either case a single flow at the beginning of the sentence usually would carry the patient through the entire sentence. In other words, even if the frequency of laryngospasm was high, its firmness was not, and the flow was generally effective.

But if the word or sound stress within the sentence was high, or if the patient had an extremely high baseline stress (a Chihuahua), the firmness of the closure might be so great that several airflows would be required within each sentence. After using this technique success-

101

fully so that the baseline stress or word or sound stress dropped, the patient might then only have to use a single flow at the beginning of the sentence.

Some patients whose stress did not drop had to continue using several flows during each sentence. The patients rightly objected to this; it virtually destroyed the rhythm of speech and was very obtrusive. For these patients I developed a technique which, although not as aesthetically pleasing as pure flow, nevertheless enabled them to speak at normal rhythms.

Basically the technique involved a change in the patient's speech. Instead of speaking normally after passive airflow, the patient spoke in a breathy fashion. The breathiness was the result of the patient's never firmly closing his vocal cords, but speaking with them perpetually open. Thus airflow was present not only before each sentence, but throughout it as well.

Admittedly this solution was less than perfect, but it was the only suitable means I could devise for treating this severe stuttering problem. Some of these patients later overcame enough of their stress to enable them gradually to give up their breathy voice and use the airflow simply at the beginning of each sentence. It must again be pointed out that the group diagnosed as severe stutterers constituted no more than about 12 percent of my patients. About half of these were able to deal successfully with their excessive stresses and ultimately acquired fluency.

26
THE CONCEPT
OF
TOTAL CURE

I VIEWED THE FIRST WEEK of therapy—the intensive phase—as an opportunity for the patient to learn quickly a new set of habits which functioned in a manner directly opposed to the old ones. It was very important to remind the patient repeatedly that the old habits had been practiced millions of times and were therefore extremely well learned and deeply entrenched. The new habit, on the other hand, even though it brought immediate fluency, possessed virtually no strength. It was no cure.

The purpose of the second phase, therefore, was to build the strength of the new habit to the point where it could compete successfully against the old habit under all conditions of stress. This process took time and extensive practice and there was no way around it.

Thus the following situation often occurred. The patient would be fluent at the end of the first week and would be required to practice daily for months afterward with no appreciable change in performance. Unlike other skills, in which practice improves the performance, thereby sustaining motivation, for my patients practice served only to strengthen the already developed skill of fluency, making the habit grow in strength so that it would not disintegrate under stress. I told patients to think of their practice as deepening a groove in their brains, with each instance of correct practice as an investment which would pay dividends in permanent fluency and lead to an eventual cure.

As I differed with my colleagues with respect to the concept of severity of stuttering, so also did I disagree with their concept of cure. Most of my patients were totally fluent after the first few days of the intensive phase of therapy: no stuttering occurred in any situation. Surely one might imagine that if a person didn't stutter he would be cured. Of course the patients didn't think so and neither would my colleagues since a relapse could occur at any time. But if I asked, "What about a patient who hadn't stuttered in ten years? Would he be cured?" the answer would invariably be "Yes. Such a long period of fluency would effectively demonstrate a cure." But then I would tell them about patients like the judge, an expert circumlocuter, a man who lived in constant fear of stuttering but who never stuttered. And I would ask them if they would consider him cured. . . .

Thus the presence of fluency does not imply a cure. A cure exists only in the mind of a speaker, not in the ears of a listener. I proposed a new definition for cure: a patient was cured, not when he didn't stutter, but when he remembered that he used to think of himself as a stutterer.

Patients were often made aware of my definition of "cure" throughout the intensive first phase of therapy. They were told that getting them fluent was absolutely no challenge at all, that a cure was not to be found in the mouth but in the mind. Cure was mental: the cured person was one who remembered when he used to stutter. Of course there could be many mini-cures. A person could, for example, remember when he used to stutter on the telephone or in front of a particular person. These situations now harbored no fear for him; he no longer ever stuttered in them; he was cured in them. But he still feared speaking to his boss or to an audience, and while he did not stutter in these situations his active fear of stuttering implied no cure.

A total cure probably takes years. Fears die slowly. Let me give a personal example. I could not swim until the age of twenty-three. I had a deathly fear of the water, had learned this fear as a youngster, and through avoidance behavior, had built it steadily to near panic as an adult.

Then I encountered a "therapist" (a lifeguard) in whom I had great confidence. Gradually, through daily practice over a period of several months, I was able to overcome my fear and relax, and I learned to swim in shallow water. Eventually the day came when I was told that I had to swim in water over my head. Having built my confidence gradually over the preceding months, I now approached this great test. With heartbeat racing I began to swim in water over my head, but I swam around the edge of the pool so that at any moment I might grab something solid should a sudden panic cause me to revert to my old behavior pattern. Fortunately I did not panic and swam in deep water.

But I was not cured. I still feared deep water, even though I was able to swim in it. And today, some sixteen years later, in sudden unexpected situations, I sometimes experience a temporary reappearance of that old fear. Although I am now an excellent swimmer I may never be completely "cured." Such is the strength of well-learned early fears.

27
ALTERED
SELF-CONCEPTS

NEAR THE END of the first week of therapy the patient
and I have a discussion of self-concept. All of us have
some idea of the kind of picture we present to the world.
From past experience we may think of ourselves as
somewhere between beautiful and ugly, intelligent and
stupid, active and lazy, etc. In large part a person's self-
concept is derived from observing other people's reactions to him.

Imagine, therefore, the self-concept of a stutterer
resulting from observing his listener's reactions. Many
stutterers report that when the first block occurs they
suddenly feel inferior to the person to whom they are
speaking. Other patients report that the shame and embarrassment of seeing the reaction of their listeners is so
painful that they shut their eyes. As a matter of fact,
stutterers frequently close their eyes during the stuttering block.

It is important for the patient to realize that a person's self-concept could exist on both a conscious and a
subconscious level. Since subconscious awareness is an

important determinant of conscious behavior, one cannot change a habit by consciously wishing to do so unless one's subconscious intent also is altered.

The patient is informed that his subconscious self-concept is that of a stutterer. When he suddenly becomes fluent, his subconscious interprets this accomplishment as a fluke, caused perhaps by some downward shift in baseline stress. In all probability the patient had known brief periods of fluency in the past, and so this newly acquired fluency for which there was some precedent would not affect the stutterer's self-concept.

But after a few weeks of fluency, the subconscious becomes "concerned." This does not fit into the ordinary picture and an attempt is made to restore the status quo, confirming the old self-image.

Suddenly, for some inexplicable reason, the patient experiences a nameless anxiety, a certain heightened tension—the cause of which he cannot fathom. It is, of course, the attempt of the subconscious to reestablish stuttering by raising baseline stress. The patient is told that the subconscious resists change and that he will not be on the road to permanent recovery unless he has fully convinced the subconscious that this fluency is, indeed, no fluke.

The patient is warned to be prepared for this test anywhere from two to six weeks after the first phase of therapy. When it does occur (it isn't by any means inevitable since some patients never experience it), he should redouble his efforts, not surrender. And shortly, usually within a week, his subconscious gives up, and he has then crossed the last major hurdle on the road to recovery.

This battle of will I recognized as one of the major stumbling blocks in some of the therapies of the past. The patient would attain fluency, thus lowering his baseline stress, and making him feel self-confident. Then his baseline stress would suddenly rise precipitously as a result of the assault of the subconscious, causing him to tense his cords and stutter. This would raise his baseline stress, and he would have a full-blown "relapse."

A young patient once said to me, "You know, Doc, it's ninety percent mental." According to my own estimate, she was a little off; it is closer to 98 percent mental.

28
THE AIRFLOW
HABIT

MOST PATIENTS ASK if they will be required to pay constant attention to the airflow for the rest of their lives. Although this prospect is certainly superior to stuttering, it is not a particularly appealing one. In response I indicate that the flow usually starts to become habitual after about sixteen weeks of practice, becoming automatic first in low-stress environments and last in very high-stress situations.

The process is much like learning to drive an automobile. At the beginning the new driver pays very careful attention to every movement of the steering wheel; after more and more driving experience, the steering movements become almost automatic, and the driver starts to focus his attention on other things. But let him approach some narrow bridge crossing, a situation with some potential stress, and he refocuses his attention consciously once again to the careful control of steering.

One patient likened the automaticity of his flow to ice-skating. When he inhaled he thought of himself lifting his foot, the exhalation was the smooth passage of his foot and skate onto the ice, and then he glided through the sentence. He imagined himself ice-skating through his sentences, gliding smoothly from one to the next, to the next. The concept was in the background of his conscious awareness; it virtually never intruded upon his thoughts—except under high stress.

Each patient developed his own technique of awareness. Some had a vague feeling of the air flowing from their mouths, others of their chest walls dropping, others of a sense of relaxation associated with the flow. Patients were encouraged to seek out their own key, a key that would tell them all was going smoothly and properly.

It was important, however, that the key be valid. One patient, for example, developed the habit of slightly lowering his head with every airflow. After about three weeks into the second phase of therapy he reported having difficulty. I ascribed this initially to a rise in baseline stress produced by his subconscious, but when I listened to his tape recordings I could not hear the flow. He assured me, however, that he was breathing properly. I doubted this, and since he lived near my office, I asked him to come in to see me.

When he first appeared and started to speak, I noticed that he was, indeed, using the airflow technique and that each flow was accompanied by the head-lowering gesture. But after about twenty minutes of conversation he spoke without the flow but continued to move his head downward at the appropriate times. When I stopped him to ask if he was still breathing properly he insisted that he was. I then recognized his problem. He was paying attention to his key and not to his flow. Thus each time he lowered his head he thought he was using the technique when, in fact, he wasn't.

It was therefore always important to make sure that whatever key the patient used for flow awareness was indeed functioning the way it was supposed to function. Flow works because it is there and not because one thinks it is there.

29
MOTIVATION

MOTIVATION, OF COURSE, is a primary requisite for learning a new and permanent airflow habit. Several techniques have been employed successfully to intensify patients' motivation, though none was as effective as in the case of a Marine sergeant on whom I was able to impose an artificial but extraordinarily high degree of motivation.

One day I received a call from an officer in the Marine Corps who said he had a sergeant in his office who was a very capable person except for his severe stuttering. Could I treat him? I arranged for an evaluation, the results of which showed excessive struggle behavior coupled with mild laryngospasms. He was an ideal candidate. There was only one proviso. I requested that he be sent to me "on orders." In other words, I was to be his commanding officer and he would have to take direct orders from me and follow them rigorously.

This new role made my task quite easy. The patient responded to my requests as direct orders. He had to use the technique at all times; he could not flinch from his duty. He was symptom-free at the end of the week and remained under orders from me for one year to build the strength of this habit. I wished I had the same power over other patients. But lacking this power I had to resort to other methods, such as contract therapy, for enhancing the motivation of my patients.

Contract Therapy. This technique was developed originally as a means for instilling motivation in people wishing to alter two well-known and undesirable oral habits: overeating and smoking. For instance, an overweight patient makes a contract with his therapist or a friend which specifies that if the patient does not lose a certain amount of weight by a certain time he will forfeit, say, a sum of money. If he attains his desired weight, he avoids the financial loss. Another example is a heavy smoker I knew who wished to rid himself of the habit of smoking. He decided to do this by first giving up smoking at the office. It was a large office, shared by many coworkers, whom he gathered together at noon one day to distribute Xerox copies of a contract in which he agreed to give anyone five dollars each time he or she caught him smoking.

For the first two weeks he was fine; the recently made contract loomed large in his conscious awareness. He was, by any standard, motivated. But one day, in a particular situation of stress, he opened his desk drawer, discovered a cigarette, and lit up. In an instant, eight people pounced on him and he was quickly relieved of forty dollars. He has not smoked in the office since then.

I have encouraged stutterers who are intensely eager to strengthen their new flow habit to make such a contract. They know full well that if they stutter they have failed to use the flow properly and may also not have slowed their first syllable. The contract which they draw with friends and family states, "A dollar a stutter, payable immediately upon demand." Of course this varies a bit with the financial condition of the patient. A young Texan I treated, with a monthly allowance from his parents of three thousand dollars, had his contract raised to ten dollars a stutter. The loss must represent a real loss.

Contract therapy, however, is not for everyone. For some, the threat of loss is counterproductive in that it raises baseline stress and serves to frustrate attempts at passive flow. For these patients another technique I call the monitor system is employed.

The Monitor System. This technique makes use of a group of people who function to remind the patient to use his technique. Whenever a monitor sees the patient stutter he makes some agreed-upon gesture such as rubbing his chin, which means, in effect, "Come on, friend, do what you know how to do." This reminder, when applied conscientiously by appointed monitors, serves to generate a continuous form of pressure which, while not as threatening as a contractual arrangement, nevertheless serves to keep the patient's level of alertness high.

A monitor may lose his effectiveness, however, by

accepting stuttering and thus reinforcing it. When this happens, it is a distinct disservice to the patient and the scene is set for the patient to "get away" with his non-fluencies. This must not be allowed to happen, and the patient is encouraged to change monitors when it does.

Visual Reminders. As I attempted to motivate patients, it became more and more apparent that a set of visual cues would be extremely effective in reminding them to attend to their techniques. To summarize the behavior I wanted my patients to maintain, I created the five-word motto, "Passive flow, soft and slow," symbolized as PFSS.

The "passive flow" and "slow" components of the motto are, of course, the basic rules. The word "soft" cautions the patient to speak softly because of the finding that stuttered syllables are often produced more loudly than fluent ones and that such unnecessary loudness produces excessive tension in the vocal cords.

With a label maker, a number of PFSS labels were made on adhesive-backed plastic material and given to each patient. The patient was instructed to paste one on his watchband, on the dashboard of his car, on his telephone, on his mirror at home—wherever he might be during the course of the day. The purpose of the PFSS labels was to act as a constant reminder for the need to practice as much as possible. The principle was, the more visual reminders, the more practice, and the more practice, the sooner the recovery.

As one might imagine, the presence of all these PFSS labels often provoked interest on the part of the patient's friends and associates. They wanted to know what they meant. This provided the patient with the opportunity to function as an educator.

The Patient as Educator. In the process of educating people on the subject of stuttering the patient covers two specific areas: how it is that someone begins to stutter, and what he or she can do about it. To help the patient with this educational task, I prepared a fifteen-minute tape recording which dealt with both of these subjects. The patient was to listen to the recording frequently so that he could familiarize himself with its subject matter and use it in his educational task.

Functioning as an educator serves four purposes: First, such education keeps the subject matter continuously in the patient's mind. Second, discussing stuttering with people often greatly reduces the stress normally present in such conversations. Third, the educating experience is a logical lead-in to the occasional request made to a listener that he or she function as a monitor. And fourth, by so educating people, the patient is helping to reduce the general misunderstanding by the public about the cause and treatment of stuttering.

The patients were instructed to "educate" a different person each day for one month, when possible. Most reported that this became a progressively easier task and that it did help reduce stress substantially. The role of

117

educator is now routinely assumed by patients as part of my treatment of adult stutterers.

The Early Morning Pep Talk. There was still another motivational device I made use of in the treatment of stuttering. A form of brainwashing, it consisted of an early morning pep talk. I had known, from my studies of hypnosis, that the subconscious is most amenable to suggestion in the morning when the patient just awakens and the "cobwebs" are still in his head. At this time each morning, the patient, in a minimal stress condition (i.e., all alone), uses the PFSS technique on each sentence of a fifteen-minute pep talk he gives himself. In this pep talk he recommits himself to the need for the calmest, most passive flows, the absolute requirement for a slowed first syllable following each flow, and the idea of a general softening of the voice.

In addition, during this time the patient considers what may be stressful for him during the upcoming day and takes this opportunity to make a formal positive statement about how well he intends to perform in these high-stress situations. He uses this technique to "set himself" for the day.

The cumulative effect of these daily pep talks has proven to be a valuable element in the motivational phase of therapy. In a sense it is clearly a form of "the power of positive thinking," possessing many of the attributes of autosuggestion. It helps reduce baseline stress and often functions as a verbal tranquilizer for the patient. It is a technique which is now routinely used by my patients.

A Public Announcement. A very large part of the fear associated with stuttering stems from the patient's unwillingness to stutter. This may sound a bit strange, but it has been shown that the fear of stuttering in a particular situation is often greater before the patient stutters in that situation than after he does so. It is as if the patient is continuously trying to hide the fact that he stutters and it is this constant attempt to avoid exposure which perpetuates the fear and thus the stuttering. But when the stutter does occur it is an announcement that he is a stutterer and thus is sometimes stress-reducing.

I decided it would be a good idea if the patient himself, instead of his stuttering, announced to the world that he was a stutterer. For this purpose a button was made which read: "I occasionally stutter—therefore I am talking slowly these days." Patients were invited to wear this button when practicing their assignments in stores, and when speaking with friends and associates. The presence of the button helped alleviate the stress associated with such confrontations. It was clearly an about-face: from an attempt to conceal to an act of revelation. One patient described the experience as "a vacuum cleaner for the mind."

Group Reinforcement. As indicated, patients were seen intensively for the first week and then given weekly

119

assignments to practice at home, make tape recordings, and send them on to me. Most of the patients complied readily with the terms of their weekly assignments. My job was to listen to their performances and determine whether they were maintaining proper technique as they practiced each of their assigned tasks. In this way I was able to monitor their performances and abort any undesirable slippage while they were in the process of strengthening their new habit.

A number of patients, however, felt somewhat isolated in this task and wished to have communication with other patients using the same technique. This was arranged when possible. And in certain large cities such as New York, Philadelphia, and Boston, groups of my patients in the second phase of therapy were established and met on a monthly basis to share their experiences. These monthly meetings provided great motivational impetus to the participants, and though I attended a few at the start, they eventually became self-sustaining. Members of each group often break up into pairs who work with each other in supportive and challenging ways. Monthly meetings, when possible, are extremely worthwhile adjuncts to the therapy program; I hope that such groups will be established and sustained in major cities throughout the country before too long.

The Hotline. A discussion of motivation would be incomplete without considering the problem of the persistent self-stresser. In a substantial number of cases I discovered that an initial period of virtually complete fluency, lasting a month or more, would be followed by increasing difficulty as the patient overreacted to a certain situation that raised his baseline stress, reawakening many of his old fears. He would now have, for example, that old trouble saying his name and would once again live in grave fear of having to do so.

The patient had earlier been instructed to call me as soon as he started to experience difficulty. My object was to prevent the build up of self-stressing to high levels. Worrying about blocks is counterproductive since it is self-defeating; I wanted the patient to substitute an analytical mode of thinking for an emotional one. If a stuttering block occurred, it was for a logical reason: he either misused the airflow or spoke the first syllable after the flow too rapidly; there were no exceptions to this. This analysis, which the patient should have performed himself but had forgotten to do because of the stress, comforted the patient, lowered his baseline stress, and reestablished his motivation to continue practicing. I have found the use of the hotline telephone another valuable adjunct to therapy. If I can speak to the patient on the telephone before his baseline stress rises significantly I can effectively counter any deterrent to motivation.

30
WORKING
WITH
YOUNG CHILDREN

I DEVELOPED A DIFFERENT technique for helping patients under the age of eleven. I found that young children do not generally bear up well in an intensive therapy program. In addition, they require much more careful monitoring of speech during the second phase of therapy. Hence, I decided to assign these young patients to qualified speech therapists who lived in the same area as the patient and who had indicated a strong desire to learn a successful method for treating stuttering. I offered to train the therapist if he or she agreed to work with the child on a regular basis for a period of six months. The therapist was free to use the method with other patients and to consult with me should problems arise.

So I arranged to see these young patients and their accompanying therapists for a four-hour intensive session. I started by explaining my orientation to the therapists and then having them observe me do therapy. I then taught them about the misuses of airflow and the seven basic stresses and observed them as they worked with the children. A tentative therapy program was laid out for the first several weeks.

I found that this technique generally worked quite well. There were, of course, differences among the patients and among the therapists. But in general most of the therapists have made appreciable progress with their patients.

Over sixty therapists have been trained to date; hundreds more will be trained in the coming years. It is clear that the most productive expenditure of time will be invested in this training program, and I hope that several of the intensively trained therapists can be recruited for this task. The goal, of course, is to eliminate the problem in all children early in their lives so that it does not have the psychologically devastating effect upon social and personal adjustment seen so painfully in adult stutterers.

123

PART III
Case Happenings

31
NOW
YOU'RE TALKING

In APRIL 1974, after I appeared on "The Today Show" to discuss my discovery of a new and seemingly valid theory of stuttering, I received a flood of requests for further information. Many of these were from individuals who subsequently came for therapy, a few of whom have already been introduced in the preceding pages. This section is devoted to several interesting patients whose case histories I call happenings because many of their symptoms and the events occurring in their treatment were totally unexpected. Indeed, some of them were treated in locations quite remote from my office, as in the following case.

Every year I charter a sailboat and cruise the waters of the Chesapeake Bay, exploring the rivers that empty from the Eastern Shore of Maryland into the bay. Parts of this shoreline are from another age, an age of quiet, relaxation, and gentleness. I cruise for about ten days and invariably emerge from these voyages refreshed.
One afternoon I approached the municipal dock of

a small village far upriver and prepared to toss a line to a black boy standing next to a piling. As I approached, it became evident he had been anticipating my action and was delighted to be able to participate in the tying up of the boat. He caught the rope smartly and with expert speed and proper use of knots made it secure to the dock. He did the same with the two other lines I tossed him.

I stepped onto the dock and congratulated him on his expert seamanship. I asked his name. And it was then I knew—the facial struggles, the loss of eye contact, the gasps. I sighed and wondered, "Should I let it pass?" I had planned to stop only for ice, intending to sail farther upriver before nightfall.

But here was this little boy (I later found out he was ten) in this rural backwater, and I knew I would probably be the only chance he might ever have. Oh, hell, I thought, I'll spend the night here. So we sat down on the dock, and I started therapy.

He was brilliant; his blocks aborted in less than five minutes. He understood everything; he was transfixed by this person who had stepped off a boat and shown him how to talk.

We worked until ten o'clock that evening. He spoke for hours and did not stutter. Could I pump enough information into him? Could I prepare him for the stresses that must inevitably occur? There was a public telephone on the dock. We practiced our phone work there, calling long-distance operators all over the country. We made speeches to imaginary classrooms; we role-played.

He left me that evening, an evening that was very special for me and perhaps a bit magical for him. He never knew my name; he never asked for it. But I sometimes wonder what happened when he went home that night. Did he maintain his fluency? And what did his parents think? How could he explain it to them? Should I have told him my name, and given him my address? Perhaps not doing so was wrong, but I gave him my best that day and he took it beautifully.

32
THE D.A. STORY

I TREATED ANOTHER bright boy, but the situation and the setting were quite different. One day, after my appearance on "The Today Show," I received a phone call from the assistant district attorney in a West Coast city. He had seen me on the program and related the following story.

Years earlier a young man, just discharged from the armed forces, found himself being evicted from his home for nonpayment of back taxes. Even though he had been offered work after his discharge he had remained unemployed and adamantly refused to pay the city the taxes on his house. On the day set for his eviction, he donned his military uniform, and holding an American flag in one hand and his two-year-old son in the other, he called upon the press to witness and photograph the eviction.

The eviction took place forcibly, photographs were taken, and the ex-serviceman sued the city for unnecessary physical violence. He later added to the suit the charge that the incident had caused his young child to begin to stutter. Now, ten years later, the case was coming to trial.

The assistant district attorney wanted to know whether the eviction episode could have caused the son's stuttering. My response was that it could. Then he asked what it might cost to treat the stuttering problem. It was impossible for me to answer that question without seeing the child.

And so it was that I flew to that city and met the assistant district attorney, who introduced me to the child, his parents, and attorneys for the plaintiff. I was told that one of the parents would be present during the evaluation. I refused, saying that I would be happy to meet with the parents afterward to discuss my findings, but that I needed an hour alone with the child to obtain the necessary information. After a brief discussion among the attorneys, my request was met and the evaluation began.

I discovered that the child's stuttering was relatively mild; that is, his laryngospasms were weak and his stress was minimal. He caught on to the use of airflow immediately and became symptom-free after about fifteen minutes. Prior to this, he had been what is generally called a severe stutterer, as his struggles were violent and frequent. Now he spoke normally. We strengthened this habit in the remaining forty-five minutes before returning to the group. The boy was obviously delighted and so was I. Together we planned a demonstration of his fluency.

131

As we approached the others we started a conversation. After he had spoken about a dozen sentences fluently, the boy's father screamed in rage and one of his attorneys uttered a profanity while the assistant district attorney roared with laughter. The boy looked absolutely bewildered. I tried to speak, but the assistant district attorney placed his hand over my mouth and, still laughing, took me by the arm and pulled me down the corridor away from this incredible scene. I was not permitted to speak to the child.

Only later did I realize that the boy's recovery had destroyed a well-planned case against the city. I shall never forget the face of that father, a mixture of astonishment and hate. I thought he would be immensely pleased by his son's performance, but greed had corrupted him, leading to the ugly exploitation of his child's affliction.

33
THE MAN
WHO STUTTERED
AND DIDN'T KNOW IT

THE NEXT HAPPENING also began with a phone call, this time from a man who said that he had stuttered as a child but had outgrown it. However, he was plagued by an involuntary violent head-twisting gesture, similar to what he had heard me describe as one of the symptoms of stuttering. He was dubious, however, that it was stuttering because it happened not only when he was speaking, but also when he merely listened; in addition, it didn't affect his speech, but preceded it. He had been to many neurologists and all the tests had proven negative. It was most often diagnosed as a "functional nervous tic," for which he was urged to seek psychotherapy. He had gone to a psychotherapist for several years, but with no success.

He was desperate. The violent head-twisting gesture was so bizarre that it put most people off. He sincerely wished to marry but no woman would sustain a relationship with him. He felt alone and frustrated. Would I see him?

He walked into my office displaying the violent gestures he had described to me over the phone. As he spoke it occurred more frequently, but it clearly happened also while he listened to me. If one merely observed him while he spoke, he would appear to be a Type II stutterer, but how could one account for the nonspeaking struggles? The behavior obeyed some of the rules of stuttering: it increased when the stress levels increased, and its frequency pattern was fairly consistent when it appeared in conjunction with speech. There was also the additional piece of evidence that he had been a stutterer as a youngster.

When he tried the airflow technique with his speech, the bizarre behavior disappeared totally. I now knew that he was a stutterer and that he was going into laryngospasm before he spoke. Furthermore, here was an individual who apparently went into largyngospasm even when he listened.

We are all familiar with the fact that many of us, when listening to others, nod our heads in agreement and often vocally indicate participation in the conversation by saying uh-huh, or making some other kind of vocal gesture. Research has shown that these gestural agreements are sometimes subvocal; that is, we may tense our vocal cords without producing sound. And that's what this man was doing. As he listened, he subvocally responded to the speaker and these responses produced laryngospasms and the head-twisting gesture. When I asked him to breathe calmly in and out of his mouth as he listened to me, his nervous tic aborted.

I treated him successfully in several sessions and he has remained symptom-free. I often refer to him as the man who stuttered and didn't know it.

34
THE SCREAMING
PROFESSOR

AMONG MY PATIENTS who never stuttered but who nevertheless were stutterers was an individual I called the "screaming professor."

When I first evaluated his speech problem, I was amazed to discover that, although he was at a distance of no more than three feet from me, he spoke as if he were speaking to a large audience in an auditorium with no public address system. He literally screamed at me but he did not stutter.

I asked him why he used this most unpleasant level of voice, a level which must surely offend everyone he spoke to. He said he was fully aware of the unpleasantness of this habit, but that he could not stop because if he did he would stutter. In fact, whenever he felt a "tightness in his throat" coming on he would speak even louder to deal with it. He had learned to do this a long time ago and it had proved a successful tactic. But now he was unhappy about it and wanted to stop.

Here is what the "screaming professor" had learned to do: Unknown to himself, he had discovered that the primary means by which speakers control the loudness of their voice is through the amount of air pressure built up in their lungs. He had discovered, in effect, that by building up a large amount of air pressure he could blast his way through any laryngospasm that might occur; thus he always spoke loudly as a preventive technique. This, of course, lowered his stress since he expected this behavior to work, and since it usually did, it became habitual.

I taught him the airflow technique, which he substituted for his "head of steam" approach. Thereafter he continued to be fluent, but now as a "soft-spoken professor."

35
THE COUGHING
STUTTERER

ANOTHER FORM OF the "head of steam" tactic as a coping device appeared as a persistent cough in an eleven-year-old child. He had started coughing about three years prior to my seeing him, following an upper respiratory infection, and had shown no remission. The child had been taken to a variety of medical specialists but no physical cause could be found. Again the parents were told that this was a nervous disorder, and again treatment by psychologists brought no relief. Having read an article in a magazine about my work with stuttering, they decided to call for an evaluation.

When I examined him I found that he did indeed cough frequently and that such coughs occurred at the beginnings of sentences or a second or two before the beginnings of sentences. The coughs occurred only when the sentences began with a vowel or with an explosive consonant (p,t,k,b,d,g).

The child was a stutterer, though he was not aware of it. He was using the cough to break through his laryngospasms. I taught him the use of airflow and quickly put an end to the problem.

36
THE SHINY
PENNY

ONE DAY I RECEIVED a call from a speech therapist in Denver who had read about my work with stutterers and had a patient who, she felt, might be a candidate for my therapy.

Her patient, she told me, was a reporter for a local newspaper and also a regional correspondent for a national weekly magazine. He had stuttered as a child, but had outgrown it. And then some fifteen years afterward he began to stutter again after he was told the serious nature of his father's illness.

This was clearly a case of high external stress creating laryngospasm that produced blocks and raised baseline stress. I asked the therapist to have the man call me so that I might listen to his speech. When he did, I discovered that he stuttered only on vowels and that, having been fluent for such a long period, he apparently had minimal stress.

He told me he would be in New York on business several weeks hence and wondered if I could see him then. I agreed to do so and told him that I believed his case might be mild. In fact, I said I would go out on a limb and bet him a shiny penny that I possibly could get somewhere with his problem. But first I would have to evaluate it.

I saw him an hour each morning for five days. His blocks aborted after ten minutes of the first hour. He remained symptom-free and on the fifth day made good on his bet and presented me with the penny.

Almost a year later, when I was in Denver consulting for the Colorado Hearing and Speech Center, I relayed a message to this man—a small envelope which contained a shiny penny, a reward for sustained fluency.

37
THERAPY
AT
37,000 FEET

WHAT DOES ONE DO when he has been practicing a therapy for stuttering which seems to work far better than any therapy in the past, and one encounters a person stuttering in a store or a restaurant? Should one go up to him and say, "Listen, brother, I know the answer, the way out of your misery. . ."? Or should one keep still, fearing that such a statement might prove to be embarrassing or impudent? This was an extremely sensitive moral dilemma for me.

If I approached the person, I might be accused of advertising myself, but if I didn't, the odds were he would probably continue stuttering. On several occasions I remember saying to myself, if he only knew how close he was—and then the proximity got the better of my reticence and, damning embarrassment and impudence, I plunged directly into my explanation of the cause of stuttering as if the person were a patient sitting in my office.

The suddenness of the approach and my apparent lack of self-consciousness usually disarmed the stutterer and he would stand or sit transfixed until the explanation was complete. If, after the explanation, he simply acknowledged it with a form of "thanks but no thanks," and proceeded along his own way, I was satisfied; I had done my job; my anxiety was reduced.

But if he wanted to know more, I told him more. I showed him the technique, for I felt that I might not ever see the person again. The memory of the boy at the dock created a sense of urgency and a desire to do as much as I could in the little time I had.

And so it was with this thought in mind that I heard a man in his mid thirties check into the ticket counter at an airport and stutter his way through the process of acquiring a seat assignment on the same plane that would carry me from the West Coast to New York.

I listened carefully and heard what I wanted to hear. When it came my turn I asked the ticket clerk for the seat next to his. I was going to do speech therapy at an altitude of 37,000 feet and I knew the time span within which I had to work: I had six hours before arrival at Kennedy Airport.

As soon as the plane lifted off the runway I began my explanation—no introduction, no statement of my background or interests, not even mention of the fact that I had heard him stutter. It was as if I knew all about him, and although he did not know it at the time, I had planned, again with my usual modesty, that this flight was going to be of considerable significance to him.

Following the explanation I plunged immediately into therapy. He showed an initial resistance which aborted as quickly as his blocks did. After practicing for about a half hour I had him test his new technique by summoning a stewardess and asking her for a magazine. He performed well and, since his stress was relatively low, he mastered the technique and practiced it without difficulty.

We were in one of those huge jumbo jets and decided to go for a walk. Our object was to strike up conversations when and where we could. He managed these well and when we finally returned to our seats he smiled for the first time and asked my name.

The rest of the trip was devoted to reinforcement of his new habit. As he wanted to continue treatment and lived in New Jersey, I referred him to a therapist there for weekly follow-up visits. His performance has continued to be excellent, vindicating my presumptuous approach.

38

THE PUBLIC
SPEAKER

THE CASE HISTORY of one patient is interesting because of what he decided to do after he became fluent. A man in his mid twenties with a relatively average form of stuttering, he responded to treatment without incident and progressed through the second phase of the therapy program with equal success.

Subsequently he called me for an appointment to discuss a personal matter. When we met he told me he had prepared a one-hour lecture dealing with what his life had been like as a stutterer—its frustrations, anxieties, dashed aspirations—together with a description of the therapy he had undergone and how it had completely changed his life and made him, as he said, "a member of the human race for the first time."

He had approached a lecture bureau with an outline of the lecture, and they were interested in setting up a lecture schedule for him. But before making final arrangements, he wanted the benefit of my reactions to his speech.

His lecture was very moving, filled with all the

heartrending experiences that beset the life of the stutterer. It was all there—the early unhappy experiences in school, the teasing, humiliation, and embarrassment, the avoidance of social situations, the nightmares over the use of the telephone, the difficulty in adolescence with peers, the dropping out of college and settling for an occupation far beneath one's level of capability. And then the therapy, the awakening of hope, the discovery and testing of fluency, and the emergence of a new self-concept. He had been reborn and wanted to share this with others.

I was delighted with the lecture and encouraged him in every way possible. I later discovered that, after giving the lecture about two dozen times, he had been offered a position as an executive trainee with a major retail store and has worked successfully in an executive position for them since then.

39
AN UNEXPECTED
ALLY

I GENERALLY TREAT two patients at a time, not only because a three-person interaction makes the therapy more dynamic, but also because practicing the airflow technique initially tends to produce hyperventilation, making it desirable for one patient to spell the other.

In the early stages of the development of my therapy program I would try to match patients on the basis of age and sex, both of which turned out to be totally unimportant variables. The only important factor in choosing suitable pairs is the magnitude of the stress level.

And so it was that on one occasion I paired a fifteen-year-old girl with a twenty-three-year-old man. They both had relatively high stress and I expected that their progress would be slow.

Sometimes, however, with the acquisition of new behavior, the patient's stress level drops precipitously, thus permitting a faster rate of progress. This is precisely what happened for the fifteen-year-old and precisely what did not happen for the twenty-three-year-old. When she was ready to face anything, he was still frightened of leaving the therapy room.

The disparity in their stress levels was now so great that I feared that one or both might be short-changed in terms of the amount and types of experiences that might be provided each of them. I expressed this concern aloud and the fifteen-year-old responded by saying, "Don't worry, Doc, I'll take care of it." And she drew up to her full five-foot-one-inch height, stared solidly up into the eyes of the six-foot-three-inch young man, and rendered a pep talk that would spur any team on to victory. Using words like guts and determination, she badgered him, embarrassed him, prodded him—in other words, she needled the daylights out of him.

When she finished it was time for lunch and she said she would go out with him and continue their discussion over lunch. But since she was doing all the talking, I wondered if he would be able to get a word in edgewise.

When they returned he was a new man. Using every technique that this mature fifteen-year-old could think of, she succeeded in substituting his new desire to perform for his old fear of stuttering. And with that came an equivalence in performance between the two which enabled them to progress rapidly. Never has a therapist had a more dynamic ally.

40
THE NONFLOWING
TORNADO

Occasionally, when I explain that it is necessary for a patient to spend a week with me in intensive therapy, he asks if it might be possible to break up the week into several shorter segments. I explain that it is not possible since a momentum is set up in the intensive therapy period that should not be broken. One patient, however, wanted the therapy so desperately but had such important business commitments that he wondered if we might not effect some sort of compromise. Could he leave my office number with his secretary so that she could reach him in the event of any emergency? In addition, mightn't we, in the later stages of the first phase, practice the therapy while he conducted business? I agreed to both requests.

On the Monday morning we started therapy, every fifteen or twenty minutes we were interrupted by an "emergency" phone call from his secretary. After two hours of this I told both of them that it was intolerable. We would have a break every ninety minutes and the secretary could phone only during the breaks. As a matter of fact, if there was any violation, I would simply take the phone off the hook. Here was a case of confused priorities if I ever saw one.

On Wednesday of that week he announced that he could no longer stay away from his business, and we left the office together. His business, I discovered, was conducted largely from the back seat of a limousine, equipped with two telephones and a short-wave radio unit as well; occasionally all three were in operation at once. At certain stops refreshments would be supplied; at others one or two men would join us in the car to conduct business. It was a traveling three-ring circus. And my requests to my patient to practice the flow technique created as much impact as the flies that smacked into the windshield as we sped along the highway that muggy July afternoon.

Oh, he was pleasant all right, but have you ever tried to get a tornado to flow passively? The flow, when he used it, worked, but he was too busy working to use it.

41
THE BOY
WHO SPOKE
ON LAST GASPS

THE FOLLOWING CASE is representative of many persons who display the same behavior. The patient appears to expel almost all the air from his lungs and then to speak two or three words on the remaining breath. The air is usually pushed out very forcefully and the patient must speak quickly before the air is totally exhausted—a process that is extremely tiring since the forceful expulsion of air requires extensive use of the abdominal muscles. The question is, Why does the patient adopt this behavior?

It is an important question because this type of patient is seen so often by speech therapists that when they hear about my technique they initially think that it produces this type of behavior. The reality, of course, is quite different. But the interesting thing is that these patients can speak, albeit fitfully, after pushing out almost all their air.

The patients themselves are usually unable to provide an explanation for their behavior. Any therapist who has seen such a patient will never forget him. The gasping for air, the rapid, staccato speech—the experience is much like watching a person in the throes of an asthma attack.

A seven-year-old boy was brought to my office with an extreme version of this problem. I could hear the forceful flow of air before every attempt to speak. Sometimes he let out so much air that he could only say one word; sometimes not even that.

His mother was frantic; she had taken him to several speech therapists but had observed no improvement. Rather, the problem seemed to be worsening and this fearsome breathing clearly frightened her.

When I suggested that the treatment for this problem would be to teach the child a new way of breathing in preparation for speaking, she thought that this indeed made a good deal of sense. But when I described the technique, indicating that the child would have to let some air out first prior to speaking, and then speak on the remaining flow, she saw no difference between this and what the boy was already doing.

I succeeded in convincing her of the difference, however. I explained that the airflow I would teach him was passive and not pushed; and the boy would let out only a little bit of air before speaking and would then speak very slowly. The technique worked for the boy immediately. The passive flow eliminated the pushed flow. The small amount of air emitted in the flow meant that the child did not have to exhale a great deal of air before speaking and thus could speak normal-length sentences.

Why the pushed flow is adopted by stutterers as a coping device is relatively easy to explain. When a person exhales almost all his air, certain receptors in his lungs tell the brain of their deflated state and stimulate an inhalation. The first step in inhalation is a marked opening of the vocal cords to allow the air in. This is accomplished by the strong contraction of a single pair of muscles, a pair of muscles that strongly opposes the laryngospasm. Thus letting out almost all the air prior to speaking is a way of successfully coping with the laryngospasm producing stuttering.

The passive airflow and slow speech is another and less tiring way of accomplishing the same end. Once the child recognized this, it was a simple matter to substitute the new behavior for the old.

42
THE SWALLOWER

A MORE UNUSUAL SYMPTOM that bears describing is seen in the patient who always swallows not only before sentences but often throughout them as well. I have had several patients whose only symptom was frequent and vigorous swallowing. The swallowing was of the Type II variety in that it preceded speech, which was invariably spoken normally. As the stress increased, sometimes two or three consecutive swallows were required before speech could be initiated. Furthermore, whereas a given stutterer might have swallowed only at the beginnings of sentences in low-stress situations, under high stress he swallowed several times within each sentence.

This form of behavior, when it occurs intermittently, is a socially acceptable coping behavior; everyone occasionally swallows before speaking. But when it increases in frequency, it becomes obvious and bizarre. Listeners do not know such patients are stuttering; they are aware only of the rather annoying behavior. The patients, of course, know they are stuttering but it makes no sense to acknowledge this to anyone.

Since the swallowing behavior is generally socially acceptable, the stress attendant upon its use is low, and the patients therefore readily learn the flow technique and substitute it for the swallowing habit.

The reason that swallowing enables the stutterer to speak is as follows. Whenever a person swallows, the vocal cords shut tightly to prevent the possibility of food being transported into the lungs. After the swallow, the vocal cords reflexively open to enable the resumption of breathing. The stutterer therefore makes us of the reflexive opening of the vocal cords after swallowing as a means for dealing with the laryngospasm.

43
TREATING PATIENTS THROUGH INTERPRETERS

SINCE THE THERAPY for stuttering is the same regardless of the language spoken, treatment can be performed effectively through an interpreter. One of the most interesting of such sessions took place with an eighteen year-old Vietnamese refugee. Two years prior to my seeing him, he had stepped on a land mine and lost his left leg. One month later his stuttering began.

Because the stuttering habit had not yet become deeply entrenched, he responded well to intensive treatment, becoming symptom-free early, and has remained so to this time.

As is customary in my therapy program, I ask patients to place a telephone call using their new technique. The phone, as has been mentioned earlier, is often an extremely high-stress situation for most stutterers. I asked the patient through his interpreter whether he had any fear of using the telephone. He indicated that the phone was not stressful for him. Only later did I find out why it wasn't. He had never used the phone in his life; he had had no access to one in his peasant village, and when he went to the city, he had no reason for calling. This was revealed when I handed him the phone and found to my amazement that he did not know what to do with it.

On another occasion I took him and his interpreter to a department store to have him practice the airflow technique, using a few stock English phrases he had learned. My plan was to explain to a few people in the store that this young Vietnamese was practicing his English and to ask them to respond briefly to him. We had done this quite a few times and it was evident that the airflow technique was working perfectly. We decided to approach one more individual with our request, and received an indifferent if not downright rude reaction. I said to the interpreter, "What a shame, everyone has been pleasant; how unfortunate to find a rude person." The young Vietnamese, seemingly unaffected by the rebuff, asked the man a question. And it was then that the man's companion spoke up saying: "I'm terribly sorry. He speaks no English."

PART IV
Suggestions for Helping Stutterers

44
FOR PARENTS
OF CHILDREN
BEGINNING TO STUTTER

ONE OF THE THINGS I have heard repeatedly from parents of stuttering children is that when their child first began to stutter, the advice of their pediatrician had been, "Do nothing, he'll outgrow it." Although three quarters of all stuttering children do outgrow their problem, it sometimes takes years, and meanwhile both the children and their parents may suffer considerably. And what about the children who do not outgrow their stuttering? How long should these parents wait before doing something?

In my opinion something should be done immediately and I have devised a simple method for helping the child that parents can use as soon as they notice nonfluencies appearing in his speech. .

Before undertaking the technique, it is important that both parents read this book so that they understand the origins and development of the stuttering block. As the role of stress cannot be exaggerated, careful attention should be given to the problem of eliminating all sources of external stress for the child. The home environment should be warm and supportive, and the parents should try to conduct themselves in as relaxed a manner as possible.

If the family environment is a calm, loving one, and if both parents can see no possible source of external stress which might affect the child adversely, then the odds are high that the child's stress is self-imposed. In this case, which is typical, the technique offered here will probably be effective in helping the child overcome his difficulty.

There are two basic speech stresses that are self-imposed in the young child: speed stress and the stress of uncertainty.

In the process of acquiring normal speech, the young child imitates the rate at which he hears others talk. And the model for this rate is usually the rate at which his parents speak. If his parents are fast talkers, the child attempts to talk fast. The parents, of course, are generally oblivious to the rate at which they speak, having acquired the facility many years earlier. But the young child, with his immature brain, finds himself hard-pressed to keep up, and his self-imposed demands for adultlike speech cause stress and produce the Airway Dilation Reflex, thus setting the stage for laryngospasm and subsequent stuttering.

Another cause of self-imposed speed stress occurs when the child begins to increase the lengths of his sentences. Most children start by communicating with single words, and then progress systematically through two- or three-word phrases to short sentences. As the number of words in a sentence increases, the speed with which each of these words is produced also increases. So, for example, if I ask an individual to say the word "the" and then the two words "the boys" and measure the durations of both "the's," I find the second shorter than the first. Thus as the child gets older and uses longer sentences, his speed increases automatically, and he may reach a condition of speed stress that produces an Airway Dilation Reflex.

The second self-imposed speech stress, called the stress of uncertainty, arises as the child attempts to use new vocabulary and grammatical forms. He becomes uncertain about which form or word is appropriate for what he wants to say, resulting in a tensing of his vocal cords that causes a laryngospasm.

When speed stress is combined with the stress of uncertainty the problem is substantially compounded. On the other hand, if the child slows his speech markedly, he usually allows himself enough time to program his speech properly and thereby eliminates almost all the stress of uncertainty. Given enough time, the child can usually deal successfully with most of the self-imposed demands for adultlike speech.

This leads to the notion that it is essential for the child who is beginning to stutter to try to speak slowly— a notion which does not sound particularly remarkable. Parents have always told stuttering children to slow down. Indeed, the fact that fully three quarters of them outgrow stuttering probably can be largely attributed to those children's ability to heed this advice. Hence, I will describe some practical suggestions for parents to help reduce the speed and uncertainty stresses under which their child appears to be operating.

The first thing parents can do is to slow down themselves. They should speak at a rate of eighty words per minute, paying particular attention to slowing every word in each sentence, with emphasis upon slowing the first word. I call speaking at this slow pace stretched speech. The parents should attempt to use stretched speech whenever they are around the child. If there are other, older children present they, too, should be encouraged to use it. In addition, the parents should attempt to use a simplified vocabulary and shorter sentences. To facilitate this, the parents might imagine that their child has just come from a foreign country and knows relatively little English, and they should speak to this child as they would to any foreigner with limited knowledge of the language—slowly and simply.

In this manner, the parents establish a model for the child to emulate, a model that will free him from stress.

The parents should identify their new speech pattern to the child as stretched speech, introducing him to the stretched-speech game. The rules of the game are as follows. Each evening Mom and Dad take turns sitting in a stretched-speech chair, and, using stretched speech, each of them alternately talking for five minutes. This becomes a nightly ritual; they have an opportunity to talk about the events of the day. The child is then encouraged to play the game. He is seated in the stretched-speech chair and told to imitate his parents' speech as he describes something that happened to him during the day. The parents may not interrupt the child, but may use appropriate hand gestures to slow down his rate if he speeds up.

If the cause of a young child's stuttering is speed or uncertainty stress, the stretched-speech game, when played consistently, will quickly eliminate the nonfluencies in the child's evening five-minute monologues. After a week or two of these performances, the child is asked to use stretched speech in other situations. For example, if he comes home excited after playing outside with his friends, and starts to stutter as he hurriedly attempts to explain what happened, he should be taken to the stretched-speech chair and urged to tell the story using stretched speech. Later on in the generalization process the chair will be eliminated and the child encouraged to talk in stretched speech whenever under stress conditions. Stretched speech therefore becomes something special for the child. It is a manner of speaking that is associated with fluency; the object is to have the child substitute stretched speech for his normal speech until his brain matures to the point where it can successfully cope with adult speech rates.

Very often parents are not sure about the precise model for stretched speech. They fear that they are not speaking slowly enough or are doing something undesirable in their performance. A simple means for achieving proper stretched speech is to select eighty-word passages from books or magazines and to practice reading each of them in one minute. No attempt should be made to change the speech in any other way; both intonation and pronunciation should remain the same.

Parents should practice eighty-word-a-minute speech several times initially and then once each day so that they become thoroughly familiar with its pace. Care should be exercised in making sure that the stretched speech involves a true slowing of all the words. Sometimes parents simply increase the length of the pauses between the words or sentences while maintaining the same rate of speech, and it is important to be on guard against making this mistake.

The stretched-speech technique has been used successfully in very young children, especially those whose nonfluencies are in the preliminary stage, that is, unaccompanied by overt struggle. It is a simple technique which I recommend for all young nonfluent children, and the results are usually immediate.

45
FOR THE
CLASSROOM TEACHER
OF YOUNG STUTTERERS

THE PURPOSE OF THIS SECTION is to offer the grade school teacher a simple procedure for reducing or possibly eliminating the child's speech problem in the classroom. Of course, one must recognize that any successful treatment involves attacking the problem on a number of fronts simultaneously. Therefore the teacher should have the cooperation of the parents and the local speech therapist, if one is involved, in treating the child. This would establish a basis for communication that would markedly enhance the effectiveness of the treatment program.

The technique I propose makes use of a well-known phenomenon in the literature on stuttering, specifically, that stutterers do not stutter when they read chorally—that is, read aloud in unison. Serving as a form of distraction, choral reading focuses the stutterer's attention away from his own speech, lowering baseline stress to the point where laryngospasm and the resultant stuttering do not occur. This choral-reading effect can be used to establish fluent speech in the classroom, and it is then possible to wean the child away from the choral dependency while maintaining his fluency. The technique, which requires very little class time each day, can be made a class project.

On a Monday the stutterer, together with five other students, reads simple materials chorally for thirty seconds. On Tuesday, using the same material, he reads for thirty seconds chorally with four students in the class. On Wednesday with three, on Thursday with two, and on Friday with one.

It is very likely that the child will achieve continued success even though the number of children with whom he reads is systematically reduced. Because of the phenomenon known as the adaptation effect, if a stutterer reads the same material repeatedly, he will have progressively less difficulty with each of the readings. So when the child is asked to read chorally the same material each day, the adaptation effect combats any possibility of increased stress associated with the reduction in size of the choral-reading group.

Of course the child does not know this; but he does know that he is meeting with continued success in a situation that had been routinely fraught with failure. This continued and somewhat unexpected success lowers his baseline stress and makes it relatively easy to begin to wean him away from the adaptation effect.

166

This is accomplished in the second week. During this time, the child is called upon to read chorally with one other child each day. Each day, however, a different passage is read. Since the child is still reading chorally and his baseline of stress is presumed to be somewhat lower, he will be likely to have continued success. If the child has some difficulty, however, the simple remedy for it is to increase the size of the choral-reading group. The usual procedure is to increase the group size by adding two readers. As soon as the child's performance is fluent, the group size may then be reduced again by one child at a time.

With the child now regularly reading with one other child it is time to begin to wean the stutterer away from the choral-reading situation. This usually can begin in the third week of the program. During this week the accompanying reader moves physically farther and farther away from the stutterer each day as they read together. Until finally, on the last day of the third week, the two speakers are reading chorally from opposite ends of the room.

On the fourth week the accompanying speaker endeavors to lower the loudness of his voice each day until finally, by the last day of that week, he is speaking barely at a level above a whisper.

On the fifth week the accompanying speaker, still talking softly, begins to leave out occasional words as he reads, leaving more and more out as the week progresses.

167

By the sixth week, the mere presence of the accompanying speaker suffices for a fluent reading performance to be achieved by the young stuttering child. Occasionally a first word of a sentence may be read chorally for support. This may be required particularly for the first word of the passage.

Two things must be borne in mind. One, after the first week, a new passage must be read each day: no adaptation is to be allowed. Second, all reading should be done at a reduced speed, especially the first syllable of each sentence. One would be wise, therefore, to choose a naturally slow-speaking child as the choral accompanier. This child may be coached briefly in reading at a rate of approximately eighty words per minute.

The above technique may be employed relatively successfully with children whose stuttering appears to be effortless. For the child with violent struggling behavior, the choral-reading technique practiced in the classroom can facilitate the progress of the child who is receiving airflow therapy from a trained professional. The child in therapy would perform the choral-reading technique as described, only each sentence he speaks would be preceded by an airflow. He would also markedly slow the first syllable after each flow.

Thus if the classroom teacher is confronted with a severely stuttering child, it would be advisable to alert the speech therapist to the airflow technique so that both might work together to apply it in the classroom situation. This would be an extremely important and worthwhile collaborative venture. Some of the deepest scars in the memories of adult stutterers are those associated with their performance in the classroom.

46
FOR SPEECH
THERAPISTS
ONLY

IN A SENSE, having a brief section devoted to information for speech therapists may strike these professionals as somewhat strange. After all, isn't the entire book precisely that? The answer, of course, is yes, but in this section my intent is to offer some cautionary advice.

I have attempted to describe my technique in detail. I recognize, however, that learning a therapeutic approach can never be accomplished through the reading of a book, regardless of how carefully it is written. There is simply no substitute for working with patients directly and observing the variety of possible interactions among patients and therapists to the airflow technique. I do not mean to suggest that the training of therapists in this technique requires a long period of internship; some therapists have been adequately trained in as little as twenty-five hours. But training definitely is required, and it is my hope that there will soon be trained therapists in each of the major cities of the country.

These individuals would act as regional resources to provide training for colleagues and thereby increase the availability of these services.

The airflow technique differs in important ways from speech therapy. As is apparent from the success of this technique, focusing on the speech problem itself has been one of the major mistakes in the treatment of stuttering. The struggle that appears so often in stuttering is not with speech but rather against a laryngospasm which has occurred just prior to speech. Therefore to work on speech is a grave mistake, and any form of therapy that does so is of dubious value.

Techniques such as bounce, pull out, and cancellation have no value when viewed within the context of the model offered in this book. Our attention, and the attention of our patients, must be constantly focused upon what they do before they speak. If they set themselves up properly, that is, use the passive flow and intend a slowed first syllable, their speech will emerge fluent. This preoccupation with preparation and disregard for speech is a major distinction between this therapy and speech therapy.

There is still another and perhaps even more important distinction. When one teaches a sound in speech therapy, one attempts to have it coarticulate, or assimilate, with its environmental sounds. This, in a sense, is what constitutes carry-over. The therapist is after the smooth transition of the newly learned sound into all phonetic contexts. In other words, it is desirable that

171

there be a mutual influence between the new sound and its neighbors.

This is precisely what is *not* wanted in the airflow technique. The therapist must be constantly alert to the importance of having the flow remain unaffected by the sound in its environment. If, for example, the patient is flowing into a lip-rounded vowel and begins to anticipate the upcoming sound too early in the flow by rounding the lips, you can be fairly certain that the patient will also be starting to tense his vocal cords for the production of that sound. The result is the strong likelihood of the occurrence of a flow that ends in laryngospasm.

Thus it is imperative that the processes of assimilation and coarticulation do not occur. Such occurrences ensure relapse, and it is important to understand that carry-over, which is so basic to speech therapy and which contains these processes, is entirely unwanted in this therapy.

It should come as no surprise, then, to discover that I often begin lectures to speech therapists with this statement, "Speech therapy does not work in the treatment of stuttering, but speech therapists, when properly trained, are probably the best people to work with stutterers."

47
FOR THE FAMILY
AND FRIENDS
OF ADULT STUTTERERS

THE ADULT STUTTERER, by definition, is a therapy failure; he has usually made two or more unsuccessful attempts to be helped by speech therapy or psychotherapy. He is often resigned to his plight and makes the best of it. So, too, do his friends and family.

Friends are often too embarrassed to bring up the subject. After all, what can they do when so many others have tried and failed? Moreover, they may have discovered that when the subject is brought up, their friend's speech worsens, and this, of course, becomes a powerful reason for never discussing it again. The logical thing is therefore to try to disregard it; and they do.

Families, while also accepting, seem to be searching for a way out. Most of my contacts with patients begin with requests for further information from a parent or a spouse who, unlike friends, understands the true dimension of the stress under which stutterers live and thus continue to be powerfully motivated to do something about it.

I propose, therefore, that both family and friends

can provide an extremely useful service by enabling the stutterer to become aware of this new development in the treatment of stuttering. There is no place for timidity and reticence when such hesitancies are stacked against the desperate conditions under which the average stutterer functions. Most adult stutterers, who have probably given up hope, should have the opportunity to consider once again the possibility of living the normal existence which is their birthright.

For those patients who have received the airflow therapy, the continued support of family and friends becomes essential. All of those truly interested in the welfare of the stutterer should read this book, particularly those sections dealing with motivation, so that they may become enlightened and constructive aids in the process. They should bear in mind that the stutterer has spent years learning to stutter and that the unlearning of it, including all the fears, will probably take at least a year or two. Helping the stutterer accomplish this is a rewarding task, freeing him from the impediment that has blighted his life.

48
FOR THE
ADULT STUTTERER
ONLY

IF YOU HAVE READ through the book up until this point, you've probably recognized yourself described several times. You appreciate your form of coping behavior and why it was developed. You know how many of the seven stresses you suffer from. Perhaps you have had a renewal of interest in the possibility of doing something about your problem. You've likely had speech therapy and/or psychotherapy and you know these simply have not worked. If they did work partially, you now understand why. The key, of course, is understanding, and what I have hoped to do in this book is to remove the mystery surrounding stuttering. You may already have experienced some reduction in your baseline stress as a result.

The treatment described may enable you to profit still further. Your stress may even be so low that you can treat yourself successfully. But that has not been the intent of this book. And if you are serious about pursuing therapy on a more formal basis, you are advised to contact a local therapist trained in the method. If you write to me I will provide a list of the names of trained therapists who practice in your area.

As you know, motivation will be your most important asset. If you feel compelled to seek therapy only because of outside pressures from family and friends, you will be approaching this experience from the wrong direction. After listening to the counsel of family and friends, you should read this book and ask yourself some truly probing questions before seeing a therapist for an evaluation. Then, with such information at hand, you can make up your own mind. The decision must always be a personal one, for the work, while not difficult, will require a high degree of determination and doggedness. In a sense, you will have to make a major commitment to restructuring your speech. Learning this new way of getting set to speak is not difficult; habituating it to all speaking situations is where the challenge lies.

Most of us take speech for granted. That even includes those who stutter. Having had this difficulty throughout life you are used to the struggling and the avoidance behaviors, even though it is often physically and psychologically exhausting. But if you have a specific goal in mind, whether it be a new career, or to seek advancement in your present one, or simply to be free of this old constraint so that you can become a new person—this goal will serve to sustain your motivation as you acquire and build the strength of your new habit.

Hundreds of adult stutterers have now received this training. The long-term success rate varies slightly from training facility to training facility, hovering between 83 and 92 percent. This high rate of success may appear startling in view of the poor results of the past. But if you will simply reread the first two parts of this book, you will understand why airflow therapy has achieved such excellent results. The therapy is based upon a theory, a theory which does a better job of accounting for stuttering than any previous theory. The therapy is a direct, logical outcome of the theory and involves not only a set of techniques, but also the patient's own understanding of how his stuttering began and why the technique is effective. This understanding is the crux of the therapy and accounts in large measure for the virtually negligible incidence of relapse.

When I explain the cause of stuttering to my adult patients the usual response is: "You know, that makes sense. It agrees with what I had always felt. I knew I wasn't crazy or neurotic." It is my sincerest hope that, having read this book, you too will feel that the contents make sense. The evidence, based upon the results of work with hundreds of people like yourself, seems to lend support to this conclusion.

Glossary

Airflow technique. A therapeutic technique which makes use of airflow as a means for preventing the occurrence of laryngospasm.

Airway Dilation Reflex. A vigorous dilation of the airway prior to a strong inhalation. The following structures dilate: the nostrils, the throat, and the vocal cords.

Anticipatory stress. The expectation of difficulty with speech.

Baseline stress. The sum total of the tension in all the muscles of the body at a given moment in time. A theoretical construct; not directly measurable.

Behavior modification. A technique for applying appropriate rewards, called reinforcers, to change behavior toward specific goals.

Clonic stuttering. Struggle associated with repetitive sound or syllable production.

Circumlocution. The act of substituting a nonfeared word for a feared one.

Conditioned reflex. A learned response to a stimulus or set of stimuli.

Contract therapy. A technique wherein a patient signs a contract to guarantee a desired performance; the penalty for failure to achieve the performance is the forfeit of a prized possession. The threat of loss is used as a motivational technique.

Coping behavior. A response to an unpleasant stimulus. Coping behaviors may be successful or unsuccessful, multiple or single, overt or covert, socially acceptable or unacceptable.

Distraction device. A stimulus that focuses a stutterer's attention away from a feared word or sound, thereby lowering stress.

Explosive sounds. The sounds p,t,k,b,d,g in English, produced by closing off the vocal tract at some point, building up air pressure behind this closure, and then releasing it with a slight explosion.

Extricatory struggle behavior. A socially unacceptable attempt at dealing with a laryngospasm.

Feedback receptors. Nerve endings located within a structure which tell the brain about conditions within that structure. For example, feedback receptors within and adjacent to the vocal cords signal the brain when a laryngospasm is present.

Flow groove. Acquiring a habit of flowing.

Inhibitory controls. The inhibiting by higher centers of the brain of the automatic responses of lower centers of the brain.

Laryngospasm. A marked tensing of the muscles within and adjacent to the vocal cords.

Larynx. Muscular and cartilage structure that lies between the throat and the windpipe. Contains the vocal cords.

Minimal stress condition. An absence of any of the stutterer's seven basic stresses. For example, speaking aloud when alone.

Passive flow. A completely relaxed exhalation following an inhalation; equivalent to the passive tidal exhalation of quiet breathing.

Prespeech posture. The posture of the speaking structures just prior to speech. Laryngospasm occurs basically as a prespeech posture.

Primary stuttering. Seemingly effortless anticipatory and/or extricatory coping behavior.

Psychosomatic disorder. A physical disorder originating in or aggravated by emotional processes.

Pushed flow. A forced exhalation achieved by active contraction of expiratory muscles.

Scanning. The habit of looking ahead for feared words. An example of anticipatory coping behavior.

Secondary stuttering. Anticipatory and/or extricatory coping behavior.

Self-stresser. An individual who responds excessively to failure or the expectation of failure; an individual who raises his baseline stress frequently and excessively.

Speed stress. Laryngospasm produced by the intent to

say a first syllable too rapidly.

Starters. A technique for keeping the vocal cords vibrating prior to the onset of speech, thereby eliminating the possibility of laryngospasm.

Stuttering block. A stress-induced laryngospasm associated with anticipatory and/or extricatory coping behavior.

Tonic stuttering. Struggle associated with fixations of the articulators on certain sounds; a tendency to prolong certain sounds with force.

Upper airway. The distance from the vocal cords to the nostrils and the lips. It includes the oral cavity, the nasal cavity, and the throat cavity.

Index

Catalog

If you are interested in a list of fine Paperback
books, covering a wide range of subjects
and interests, send your name and address,
requesting your free catalog, to:

McGraw-Hill Paperbacks
1221 Avenue of Americas
New York, N. Y. 10020